the
Natural
guide to
women's
health

'Why can't a woman be more like a man?' asked an exasperated Professor Higgins in *My Fair Lady*, a question that must hover at the back of many a man's mind at some time. The simple answer is that a woman is programmed by her hormones not only to experience certain aspects of life differently from men but also to feel and be different. Even if her personality and the expectations and pressures of modern life sometimes incline her behaviour to what is more traditionally considered 'male', these differences are always there and have a powerful influence on her health and well-being.

Twenty-first-century woman is knowledgeable about her body and wants the best treatment – medical or natural or both – for 'gynae' conditions. But every woman is different, so the 'best' calls for a personalised treatment package.

Women today also insist on informed choice; they want to know the pros and cons of each treatment, how to combine treatments safely, and what to do in what order. Such information is often hard to come by, and some doctors remain resistant to cooperative decision-making. Hence the need for *The Natural Guide to Women's Health*.

Penny Stanway's expert, up-to-the-minute and broad-ranging advice empowers a woman to make sensible decisions about her gynae health and well-being, whether this involves lifestyle changes to minimise the risk of later problems, choosing how to treat herself, or understanding what a doctor can do and knowing when to give the go-ahead. An invaluable 'symptom sorter' details the most likely causes of each problem, enabling a woman to assess her situation intelligently and without undue anxiety.

The Natural Guide to Women's Health is an indispensable handbook for women of all ages, destined to become a classic.

Dr Penny Stanway has worked in general practice, research and paediatrics, advises a major self-help group, and is an experienced radio and TV broadcaster. She is also health columnist for *Woman's Weekly* and a bestselling author. Her books include *Natural Well Woman, LifeLight, The Feel Good Facelift, Healing Foods for Common Ailments, First Baby After 30...or 40?, New Guide to Pregnancy and Babycare, Breast is Best, Coping with your Preterm Baby, Good Food for Kids* and *The Complete Guide to Child Health*. She has contributed to several medical encyclopaedias, and is medical editor of the popular partwork *Aromatherapy and Natural Health* and chief medical editor of the *Reader's Digest's Curing Everyday Ailments the Natural Way*.

the *Natural* guide to women's health

natural and medical solutions
for gynaecological ailments

Dr Penny Stanway

Kyle Cathie Limited

Disclaimer

The information in this book is not intended to take the place of personalised advice from your general practitioner or gynaecologist. Please consult your doctor if worrying or persistent symptoms occur.

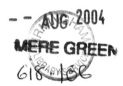

First published in Great Britain in 2003 by
Kyle Cathie Limited
122 Arlington Road
London NW1 7HP
general.enquiries@kyle-cathie.com
www.kylecathie.com

ISBN 1 85626 464 5

Project editor Caroline Taggart
Design by Robert Updegraff
Copy editor Anne Newman
Editorial assistant Vicki Murrell
Production by Sha Huxtable
Index by Alex Corrin

Printed and bound in Great Britain by Biddles Ltd, Guildford

contents

Vulva and vagina   167

Lump in vulva or vagina; sore, itchy vulva and/or vagina, perhaps with a vaginal discharge; dry vagina and vulva; bacterial vaginosis; candida infection; vulva cancer.

Pelvis   184

Pelvic pain, pelvic inflammatory disease.

Sex   191

Painful sex, low sex drive or poor sexual arousal.

Sexually transmitted infections   199

Chlamydia infection, gonorrhoea, HPV infection, hepatitis B and C, herpes infection, trichomonas infection, HIV infection and AIDS.

Menopause   215

Hot flushes, night sweats, and other menopausal signs; post-menopausal vaginal bleeding; early menopause.

Non-gynae conditions with gynae side effects or links   223

Cystitis; leaking (incontinence); osteoporosis; anaemia; overweight and obesity; binge-eating, compulsive overeating, and bulimia; anorexia; irritable bowel syndrome.

Other conditions with gynae links   248

Acne, asthma, autoimmune diseases, chronic fatigue syndrome, gluten sensitivity (intolerance), joint and muscle problems, migraine, overactive thyroid, underactive thyroid.

part three - natural cures   253

Healthy diet, foods, nutrients and gynae disorders; exercise; stress management; heat, cold and hydrotherapy; herbal remedies; aromatherapy; light

part four - what doctors can do   293

Tests and investigations, prescribed drugs, surgery, radiotherapy.

Acknowledgements

With grateful thanks to the many women who have told me their 'gynae' stories; to my colleagues in orthodox and complementary health care whose expertise and treatment of people as individuals have inspired me; to the researchers whose findings have illuminated my understanding; and to Caroline Taggart, my editor, for her good sense, enthusiasm and encouragement, and her assistant, Vicki Murrell, for her patience and hard work.

Introduction

There's been an explosion of interest in recent years in making lifestyle changes and using complementary treatments to improve our health and, as women, we are perfectly comfortable, most of the time, about doing this alongside any necessary medical treatment. Yet many of us opt out of this positive health model when it comes to gynaecological problems. The question is, why we are so passive about our 'gynae' health?

Perhaps it's because we've been conditioned by a paternalistic healthcare system into thinking that doctors always know best about this area of our life. Perhaps we have unfinished emotional business that prevents us from taking responsibility for the most intimate parts of our body. For example, we might at some level be frightened of the power our reproductive system has over our life; angry about how work, money and housing influence our plans for having babies; anxious about sex and relationships; or emotionally distanced from our physical femininity. Or perhaps we're simply too selfless – trying to do the very best for our partners' and children's health while doing less than the best when it comes to our own.

Instead of opting out of active involvement with our gynae health care, we need to create a set of strategies that includes the positive behaviours we embrace in other areas of health. We should also take the time to learn more about the choice of medical treatments, since despite the fact that they're often helpful, sometimes essential and occasionally life-saving – they often have side effects, don't always provide a long-term solution, tend to be over used and expensive, and in many cases are evolving so rapidly that we can't rely on old information. We owe it to ourselves to be more aware.

The Natural Guide to Women's Health aims to let some light and air in on gynaecology so as to remove it from its 'shroud of mystery'. The book describes and explains any problems that might arise with your breasts, vagina, womb, ovaries, sex-hormone glands or other parts of your reproductive system, and helps you choose a well balanced approach to treating each ailment. There's information on simple lifestyle changes which help the body to heal itself and stay well, including eating a healthy diet, keeping to an appropriate weight, getting the right amount of exercise, being a non-smoker and managing life's stresses effectively. There's guidance on safe and gentle complementary treatments that are easy to do at home, such as exercise therapies, hydrotherapy, aromatherapy and herbal remedies. Lastly, there's guidance on medical options, their pros and cons, and when it's wise to see the doctor.

Like women throughout the ages, women today often laugh and cry together over their experiences with periods, sex and relationships, pregnancy, childbirth, breastfeeding, the menopause and ageing. But the flood of information from medical research, health books, self-help groups, health charities, and the Internet – along with knowledge of how women cared for their health in the past – means there is much more need today than ever before to share our challenges and strategies. *The Natural Guide to Women's Health* is a celebration of women's health solutions that will empower you to start choosing for yourself so that, whatever your gynae problem, you'll be better equipped to create the treatment package that suits you best. Now it's over to you ... and I wish you many blessings on your journey

part one / a woman's body

'Why can't a woman be more like a man?' asked an exasperated Professor Henry Higgins in the musical *My Fair Lady*, a question I suspect hovers at the back of many a man's mind at some time or another. The answer is that a woman is programmed by her sex chromosomes, reproductive system and sex hormones not only to experience certain aspects of life differently but also to feel and to be different. Her body's influence is always there, even if her personality and the expectations and pressures of modern life make her behaviour more 'male' than her mother's or grandmother's might have been.

This said, many of us know very little about our 'women's bits' and even less about how our lifestyle can affect our gynaecological health. The result is a plethora of gynae disorders, and a groaning over dependence on drugs and surgery. This section provides information about your body that will hopefully empower you to manage your gynaecological health care in a reliable, knowledgeable and practical way.

sex chromosomes

At conception a tiny sperm joins a very slightly larger egg to form the single cell that's the earliest stage of a new life. This cell contains 46 chromosomes – 23 of which come from the sperm and 23 from the egg. The chromosomes carry the new individual's genetic blueprint and each one is a coil of two intertwined strands of DNA (deoxyribonucleic acid). These two strands are linked in many places – so if a whole chromosome were stretched out, it would look like a spiral ladder – and the full set of chromosomes in a newly fertilised egg contains well over three billion links. Scientists describe these links as 'letters' of the genetic code. The precise sequence of all the links determines your genetic code and, while each person's code is different (unless they are an identical twin or other 'clone'), the difference between one person's code and anyone else's is only represented by about 3 million links.

A gene is a small length of a chromosome and each gene contains a number of links. (One gene involved in the occurrence of diabetes, for example, contains around 100,000.) Each of our body's 100 million, million cells (except eggs and sperm) contains a full set of genes – which means at least 38,000 (though some scientists suspect it may be up to 115,000). These determine a baby's development, growth and characteristics, as well as influencing the activity of every body cell.

Two of a newly fertilised egg's 46 chromosomes are called sex chromosomes and these determine gender. One comes from the egg, the other from the sperm and each is either X- or Y-shaped. Sperms contain one 'X' or one 'Y', but eggs are 'X-rated' - containing only one 'X'. So the two sex chromosomes in the newly fertilised egg are either XX or XY. If they are XX, the baby will be female, and if XY, male. Very rarely, other combinations occur.

All the cells that develop from a female baby's first cell contain two Xs – with the exception of her eggs, which (like her mother's) contain only one. The XX pair not only issue instructions that make her reproductive system female but also influence every other part of her body.

reproductive system

Although the average Western woman only ever has one or two babies, her reproductive system affects her life and health in very important ways. It consists of the following:

Breasts – these contain fat, milk glands and milk ducts.

Vulva – this stretches from the hairy pubic area to the perineum (the area between the vagina and the anus). The vulva has outer and inner folds called labia (lips); interestingly enough, these have the same developmental origins as a man's scrotum. The labia surround the clitoris (in the front of the vulva), the opening of the urethra (urine passage, in the middle) and the opening of the vagina (at the back).

Clitoris – this is a main source of sexual pleasure. It has the same developmental origins as a man's penis, and in some women, according to recent discoveries, it contains even more tissue that swells during sexual arousal (erectile tissue) than does a penis.

You can feel and see two of its parts. One is the tip, covered by a small hood-shaped fold (like a man's foreskin) where the inner labia join at the front of the vulva. The other is a shaft the size of a short thin pencil, leading from the tip forwards over the front surface of the pubic bone, to which it's attached. Many people don't realise that the clitoris extends into the labia, around the urethra and the opening of the vagina, and into the front wall of the vagina – where it includes the particularly sensitive G-spot. Glands in the erectile tissue around the urethra make a fluid that enters the urethra during sexual arousal and in some women is ejaculated during orgasm.

Vagina – this leads from the vulva to the cervix and is about 8-10cm (3-4in) long – longer when sexually aroused. Most girls still have a thin membrane (hymen) across the opening in the vulva when they begin menstruating, though there's an outlet for the menstrual flow. The vagina and cervix make moisture, and production of this moisture increases at puberty, during sexual arousal, during pregnancy, and if a woman takes the combined contraceptive Pill or some other source of oestrogen.

Cervix – this is the neck of the womb and it protrudes into the upper vagina. You can probably feel your cervix if you crouch and put a finger deep in your vagina: it feels firm and has a dimpled middle.

Womb (uterus) – this is a hollow, muscular, pear-sized organ, with a lining (endometrium) which usually thickens then breaks down about once a month. The resulting menstrual blood flow – or period – contains womb-lining cells and blood. In pregnancy the womb contains and nourishes the unborn baby.

Fallopian tubes – two fine tubes that each lead from the abdominal cavity, near an ovary, into the womb. They contain thousands of tiny 'hairs' that waft an egg from the ovary into the womb each month.

Ovaries – two almond-shaped but walnut-sized structures, one each side of the pelvic cavity. They produce oestrogen, progesterone and testosterone and contain eggs, many of which start ripening but only one of which is released each month at ovulation. The ovaries usually take it in turns to ovulate .

We start life with around a million immature eggs but the number dwindles due to natural wastage so that by the time periods begin, we have only around 250,000. From then on hundreds are lost in each menstrual cycle. This is partly because of continuing natural wastage of immature eggs and partly because, while several eggs start maturing in each cycle, only one ripens fully and the rest are then destroyed. From around the age of 37 we lose eggs twice as fast. By 45, we have so few we are less likely to ovulate, so our periods may become irregular. When only around a thousand remain, we have our menopause.

The above names are the 'proper' ones for the various parts of a woman's reproductive system. However, they have many other names, some of them a lot more familiar. For example there are common names such as womb (uterus) and tits and boobies (breasts); names associated with embarrassment or ignorance, such as 'down there' (vulva and vagina); and names from other cultures, such as the Hindi yoni and poonani (vulva and vagina). There are also names with a sexual connotation, such as pussy (vulva); others with a sexual and sometimes derisory connotation, such as cunt (vagina); and, perhaps, pet or private names personal to us and to our partner or children.

sex hormones

A hormone is a powerful substance produced by an endocrine gland – a gland that releases its contents directly into the bloodstream. This explains why hormones can affect hormone-sensitive cells all over the body. When a hormone reaches such cells, tiny amounts – or molecules – of it become attached to cell receptors. These are minute structures found on the surface or in the nucleus of a cell, which are able to receive that particular hormone. When hormone molecules 'lock on' to a cell's receptors they make the cell behave in a certain way. For example, when oestrogen molecules lock on to oestrogen receptors on breast or womb-lining cells, they encourage these cells to multiply, so that the breasts swell and the womb lining thickens.

Hormone molecules lock on to empty receptors but once these are filled, a cell 'expresses' (creates) more. So the hormone's effect becomes increasingly powerful. Our sensitivity to a hormone depends partly on how much of it is circulating in the blood and partly on how many receptors our cells express. Hormone receptors are present in a surprising variety of cells; oestrogen receptors, for example, are present in brain and bone cells as well as in breast and womb-lining cells.

Many hormones, including adrenaline, insulin and thyroxine, influence our reproductive system, but some are specifically called sex hormones because of their powerful effects on the reproductive system. Sex hormones are made by the hypothalamus, pituitary and adrenal glands, and – although many people don't realise it – by the ovaries, fat cells, and, in a pregnant woman, the placenta.

sex hormones

- **Gonadotrophin-releasing hormone (GnRH)** – this is made by the hypothalamus (in the brain) and stimulates the pituitary gland (just below the brain) to produce ovary-stimulating hormones, or gonadotrophins (see below). Confusingly, GnRH has two other names: gonadorelin and luteinising-hormone-releasing hormone.

- **Gonadotrophins (ovary-stimulating hormones)** – these two hormones (follicle-stimulating hormone and luteinising hormone) are so-called because they stimulate the female gonads – in other words, the ovaries.

Follicle-stimulating hormone (FSH) stimulates 10-20 eggs to mature, or 'ripen', in the ovaries in the first half of the menstrual cycle. Each ripens in a little cavity called a follicle. The ripening eggs all produce oestrogen but before long the one that produces the most stops the others ripening fully. The level of FSH peaks before this egg leaves the ovary (an event called ovulation) then dips for the rest of the menstrual cycle.

Luteinising hormone (LH) helps to trigger ovulation then, in the second half of the menstrual cycle, stimulates the development of the corpus luteum, a temporary yellow gland that grows in the follicle vacated at ovulation. The corpus luteum produces two hormones – progesterone and oestrogen. The level of LH peaks before ovulation then remains high until just before the period.

Oestrogen – this hormone stimulates eggs to ripen; womb-lining and womb muscle cells to multiply; milk ducts in the breasts to grow; the fallopian tubes to receive an egg and the vagina and cervix to produce moisture. It also helps regulate the production of ovary-stimulating hormones (FSH and LH) and prolactin by the pituitary and tends to make us alert and decisive.

Oestradiol is the strongest or most 'oestrogenic' type of oestrogen, while oestrone is the weakest. Although oestrogens are often called female sex hormones, men have small but significant amounts too. Conversely, women have small but important amounts of 'male' hormones (androgens) such as testosterone. Indeed, oestrogen is made from testosterone and other androgens.

Oestrogens come from three places:

• Ovaries: oestradiol is made by cells within (and around) the follicles containing the ripening eggs in the first half of the menstrual cycle and by the corpus luteum after ovulation, in the second half of the cycle. Before ovulation the level of oestradiol is six times that just before a period.

• Fat cells: oestrone is made from testosterone with the help of an enzyme called aromatase.

• Placenta: oestradiol and oestrone are made from an androgen called DHEA (dehydroepiandrosterone, from the adrenals).

Progesterone – this hormone is made from cholesterol by the ovaries (especially by the corpus luteum, see page 21, in the second half of the menstrual cycle), by the adrenal glands and by the placenta. It relaxes 'involuntary' muscles (those usually outside our conscious control); lifts the mood; raises body temperature by around half a degree Centigrade and thickens the womb lining in preparation for pregnancy. It also tends to make us relaxed and calm.

Oxytocin – this hormone is made by the hypothalamus but released from the pituitary, and helps to stimulate womb contractions during menstruation, sexual breast play, orgasm, labour and breastfeeding.

Prolactin – this hormone, made by the pituitary and placenta,stimulates the production of progesterone by the corpus luteum and of milk by the breasts when breastfeeding.

Testosterone – this hormone is made from progesterone by the ovaries and adrenals. One of its actions in women is to boost sex drive.

Pregnancy hormones – these are made by the placenta and include chorionic gonadotrophins, placental lactogen, oestrogen and progesterone.

the 'conductors'

If hormones are the 'players' in the 'orchestra', then the hypothalamus in the brain and the pituitary attached to the base of the brain, are the 'conductors'. These two small hormone-producing glands influence the hormone production of all the other hormone-producing glands according to the environment inside and outside our body, so as to keep us 'in tune', or well.

The hypothalamus has receptors that are sensitive to the levels of sex and stress hormones and 'feel-good' hormone-like substances called endorphins in the blood. It also receives feedback about other body functions, body weight, physical activity, light level and some other external factors. The hypothalamus responds to this information by:

• varying its oxytocin production.

• producing releasing hormones that enable the pituitary to adjust its output of ovary-stimulating hormones, and other hormones, many of which affect the reproductive system.

• influencing the production by the nearby pineal gland of a neurotransmitter (nerve message carrier) called serotonin; this is produced by day under the influence of bright light and affects sexual behaviour, reproduction, appetite and mood. The hypothalamus also controls the production by the pineal at night of a hormone called melatonin.

what 'women's bits' do

Our sex chromosomes, reproductive organs and sex hormones affect us at every stage of our life.

infancy

Girls are often born with tiny breast swellings that if squeezed very gently may produce a drop or two of milk. This is because a baby girl is exposed – immediately before birth and via the placenta – to her mother's rising levels of breast-growth and breast-milk stimulating hormones. However, the effects of these hormones wear off soon after birth, and a girl's breasts then stay relatively flat until puberty.

A girl is born with her lifetime's stock of eggs in her ovaries.

puberty

Puberty occurs when the hypothalamus and pituitary produce enough sex hormones to kick-start the body into reproductive mode. In the average girl her pelvis starts widening, and her shape starts becoming more obviously female from 9-10. This is partly due to oestrogen, which makes fat accumulate in the breasts and over the hips and thighs. At around 10-11, her nipples start to enlarge and pubic hair begins to grow; armpit hair comes a year or so later. Breasts continue growing during the teens as fat collects between the networks of milk ducts and tiny, immature milk glands.

Around 95 per cent of girls experience their first period between the ages of 11 and 15, but it can be perfectly normal to begin menstruating at nine or even younger especially if a girl is unusually heavy, or at 15 or over if she is unusually light. The average age in westernised countries is 12½. Body weight and fat are the main predictors of the timing of a girl's first period, since most girls start to menstruate when they reach 42-52kg (92-114lb) – the exact weight depending on their height and on when their body fat accounts for 17 per cent of their weight.

With the onset of menstruation, ovary-stimulating hormones empower the ovaries to begin their cyclical production of oestrogen and progesterone. Some girls ovulate two weeks before their first period, others not for some months or even years after starting their periods. Without ovulation, periods are often irregular.

After puberty the particular levels and balance of sex hormones in a girl or woman maintain a relatively high pitch to the voice, very little body hair (other than in the armpits and on the pubis) and relatively soft and smooth skin compared with those of older teenage boys and men.

A young woman's shape helps to make her sexually attractive. So too does her natural scent: this comes partly from substances called pheromones that are produced in the armpits and by the scalp, and are sensed only unconsciously. At the same time, most girls become increasingly attracted to the opposite sex.

menstrual cycles and periods

A 'menstrual cycle' lasts between 25 and 35 days. Thirty days is the average, although 21 days can be normal and in any one woman it's usually about the same each month. Women who eat a vegetarian or other high-fibre diet tend to have longer cycles.

Normally no egg is fertilised so, when the body realises there's no pregnancy, the hormone balance changes, making the womb lining disintegrate and leave the womb as the menstrual flow or 'period'. Periods stop when a woman is pregnant and return some months after childbirth (perhaps longer if she breastfeeds frequently). They can also stop or become irregular for other reasons such as taking the Pill, losing too much weight and exercising too much.

The four parts of the cycle

1 Egg ripening and womb preparation

The pituitary responds to the sudden fall in the levels of oestrogen and progesterone at the end of the previous cycle by producing follicle stimulating hormone. This stimulates eggs to start maturing (ripening) and the womb lining, which is only 1mm (around $1/20$ in) thick after a period, to start thickening so that it's ready to receive a fertilised egg. The oestrogen level starts low, then rises to a peak nine times greater just before ovulation; this triggers a surge of follicle-stimulating hormone, and a dramatic surge of luteinising hormone – which triggers ovulation. Progesterone and testosterone levels remain relatively low, though begin to rise just before ovulation.

This 'follicular' phase of the ovary and 'proliferative' phase of the womb normally lasts for 10 -16 days and is accompanied by a ten fold increase in the amount of moisture produced by the cervix; this 'mucus' also becomes clearer and less elastic.

2 Ovulation (egg release)

One egg, occasionally two, ripens fully, then leaves the ovary and enters the nearby fallopian tube, where it's wafted to the womb. Progesterone, testosterone and endorphin levels peak at ovulation; the relatively high testosterone and endorphins boost sex drive to encourage sex and fertilisation. This is followed by a dip in the oestrogen level.

This 'ovulatory' phase lasts from one to three days (36 hours on average).

3 Development of the corpus luteum, and continued preparation of the womb lining

The departed egg leaves an empty follicle in which the corpus luteum develops. The oestrogen level dips after ovulation, but the corpus luteum (which is 1–2cm or ⅖–⅘ inch wide) then starts to produce oestrogen as well as a large amount of progesterone for around eight to nine days. Oestrogen peaks again at the beginning of the fourth week of the cycle, though not as much as before ovulation. Progesterone peaks too, reaching a much higher level than before ovulation. The amount of moisture produced by the cervix decreases markedly about 48 hours after ovulation, because the high progesterone level counteracts oestrogen's moisture-stimulating effects. Progesterone makes the womb lining thicken to around 8mm (over ¼in), and produce large amounts of a sweet carbohydrate called glycogen, ready to nourish a fertilised egg. It also switches off luteinising hormone production.

This 'luteal' phase of the ovary and 'progestational' or 'secretory' phase of the womb lasts from about 12 - 14 days. If no egg is fertilised, progesterone and oestrogen levels dip and scar-like tissue replaces the corpus luteum.

4 Period

The womb lining breaks down and its cells, along with blood, are shed as the menstrual flow. This is the 'menstrual' phase or 'period' and normally lasts from three to eight days (four to five on average). Strictly speaking, it should be classed as part of the follicular phase, since egg ripening begins during a period.

Why we have so many periods

If a woman starts periods at 13, continues till 51, doesn't use hormonal contraception, has two children, and breastfeeds in such a way that she doesn't ovulate for six months after each one, she will have around 426 periods in her lifetime, almost all of them ovulatory.

Most women think that having periods virtually all their reproductive life is normal. But this is only because we have effective contraception, and few children.

Only 100 years ago, the average woman bore six to eight children and spent most of her reproductive life either pregnant or breastfeeding, so that she only ever had around 40 periods. The same is true today among some groups of people – certain tribes in Namibia and Botswana, for example.

This is extremely different from our experience. More to the point, repeated monthly stimulation of the reproductive system by continuous menstrual cycles can encourage several gynae disorders (see page 91). This is why some doctors believe it's a good idea to suppress periods. A new brand of contraceptive Pill (Seasonale, due to be passed in the USA by the Food and Drug Administration by early 2003), supplies hormones to be taken continuously for 12 weeks, followed by seven inactive pills to allow bleeding – causing only four 'periods' a year. Contraceptive hormone injections eventually stop periods in most women too. However, critics warn that taking sex hormones for any purpose can have side effects and believe the risks of taking hormones at all, let alone continuously for three months at a time, aren't worth any potential benefits.

did you know?

- The volume of the average normal menstrual flow is 2–5 tablespoons.

- The average woman spends six years menstruating if she has two pregnancies.

- The average woman uses 22 pads or tampons during a period.

- Some of the more popular names for periods include 'monthlies', 'coming on', 'the curse', 'having the painters and decorators in', 'on the rags', 'the blob', 'riding the crimson wave' and 'Liverpool playing at home'.

pregnancy and birth

Now the body changes yet again. The corpus luteum continues to produce progesterone and oestrogen to enable the growth of the womb and placenta. These hormones, together with hormones from the placenta and pituitary, cause the breasts to enlarge as their milk glands develop. They also make the pelvic joints more flexible, in preparation for childbirth. When the baby signals it's ready to be born, the cervix softens and gets ready to expand. Then the first of the three stages of labour begins, with oxytocin from the pituitary making the womb contract rhythmically. These contractions become stronger and more frequent, gradually opening the cervix. When it's wide open, with a smooth rim, the second stage begins, with contractions that push the baby out of the womb. Last comes the third stage, in which the placenta separates from the womb and leaves the vagina.

Over the next couple of days, the breasts produce colostrum – early milk that's full of nutrients and protective factors; this then changes to become 'mature' milk, and prolactin and oxytocin from the pituitary enable a woman to make milk and let it down to her baby. Over several weeks the womb gradually returns to its pre-pregnancy size.

the menopause and later life

This marks the end of a woman's natural reproductive life and happens when she has her last period, which for the average Western woman is between the ages of 45 and 55. Sometimes periods stop abruptly or become more frequent but more often they become gradually more widely spaced. In the years leading up to her menopause, a woman becomes increasingly less likely to ovulate each month. Her levels of oestrogen and progesterone fall, and her level of follicle stimulating hormone rises. The timing depends mainly on how many eggs remain in the ovaries, and is most likely to be when this falls to around a thousand. After the menopause, sex hormone levels fall further and a woman enters the next stage of her life.

This is the time when menstrual cycles, pregnancy and breastfeeding are over and any children still at home will probably soon fly the nest. Some women help with grandchildren, some go on working and some retire, see the world, learn new skills or develop existing ones. Good health is a particular bonus because the average woman today lives much longer after her menopause than did her grandmother's or even her mother's generation.

`gyn-ecology'

Let's play with words. Let's imagine that the word gynecology (spelt the American way) no longer means the study of diseases of women. Suppose instead that it means the study of the environment ('ecology') outside and inside a woman's body and of how various environmental factors can influence her health. Such factors range from hormone and neurotransmitter levels, to immunity, light, laughter, food, exercise and sanitary protection. An awareness of their effects is important since then, as we'll see in Part Two, you can learn how to manipulate them in order to help treat gynae health problems or even to prevent them in the first place.

hormones and prostaglandins

Hormones from the pineal, thyroid, parathyroids, pancreas, adrenals and ovaries affect every part of the body, including the brain, breasts, ovaries, womb, cervix, vagina and vulva. Many lifestyle and other factors influence their production, release and efficiency, including diet, weight, exercise, light, dark, stress and sleep. While the sex hormone levels fluctuate with the menstrual cycle and various stages of a woman's life, most other hormone levels fluctuate on a diurnal (24-hour) cycle and their day-to-day levels are fairly constant. This is because they are monitored by the hypothalamus, which instructs the pituitary to increase, decrease or continue its stimulation of the various glands as necessary. Disturbances of the level or availability of hormones such as cortisol, noradrenaline and adrenaline (from the adrenal gland) and thyroxine (from the thyroid gland) can cause gynae problems, as can insensitivity of cells to any of these hormones. For example, thyroxine helps the liver to break down excess oestrogen, which means that an underactive thyroid can raise the oestrogen level. Gynae problems can also arise from an imbalance of oestrogen and progesterone (see 'Oestrogen dominance', page 89, and 'Oestrogen deficiency', page 93).

Prostaglandins are hormone-like substances made from omega-3 and omega-6 fatty acids in many parts of the body. They act locally and getting a good balance of the two main types of prostaglandins is important to gynae health. One reason for this is that it helps prevent problems such as inflammation (in the womb muscle, for example, where it causes period pain). The balance depends partly on our age and health, and partly on the proportions and quantities of omega-3 and omega-6 fatty acids in our diet. Many of us eat an unhealthily high proportion of omega-6s because of having a lot of omega-6-containing vegetable oils and margarine in our diet and a lack of foods containing omega-3s (see A Healthy Diet, page 256).

immunity

The various components of the immune system – including white cells, lymph nodes ('glands'), antibodies and substances called cytokines – help to protect against infections, including those in the vagina, womb, pelvis and breasts. Many ordinary lifestyle factors influence our immunity, including diet, stress, sleep, light, dark, exercise and the way that we breathe. Occasionally a trigger, such as raised levels of stress hormones or too much bright light, makes some antibodies misbehave and cause an autoimmune disease (sometimes inaccurately called a 'self-allergic' disease). This means they attack certain parts of the body instead of protecting them. Lupus is one example and if untreated this can cause repeated miscarriage; another is Sjögren's syndrome, which can make the vulva and vagina abnormally dry.

nervous system

Your nervous system – brain, spinal cord and 'peripheral' nerves – is vital to good gynae health because it influences sex-hormone glands and other parts of the reproductive system. Its messages are passed between nerve fibres by substances called neurotransmitters. Some act locally; others, such as adrenaline and noradrenaline, travel in the blood to affect far flung organs (which is why they are also called hormones). The best known neurotransmitters are serotonin (5HT or 5-hydroxytryptamine made in the brain, the digestive system, and the blood's platelets) noradrenaline (made by the adrenal glands and some nerve endings) and adrenaline (made by the adrenals). Others include dopamine, 'feel-good' endorphins, enkephalins, glutamate, and GABA (gamma-aminobutyric acid).

Your health and wellbeing and your diet and other lifestyle factors all affect your levels of neurotransmitters, which is partly why they are so important to gynae health.

the links between the nervous, immune and endocrine systems

These systems are very closely inter-related, so neurotransmitters, hormones and immune factors often influence each other.

For example:

• Alterations in neurotransmitter levels associated with anxiety and depression can affect the balance of sex hormones and thereby influence ovulation, periods, sexual arousal, fertility, childbirth and breastfeeding.

• Progesterone reduces the immune response to an unborn baby (which is a 'foreign' object), so preventing a woman's body from rejecting her baby.

• Oestrogen produced by the maturing egg stimulates the surge of luteinising hormone (LH) needed for ovulation.

• Certain cytokines – substances involved with our immune response – trigger ovulation by stimulating the ovary's progesterone and prostaglandin production.

• Certain other cytokines, produced during severe infection or illness, delay or prevent ovulation by reducing LH release, so ensuring that pregnancy doesn't begin at an unfavourable time.

food, drink and body weight

A good diet and efficient digestion are vital if we are to absorb enough nutrients to optimise gynae health. The three main dietary problems in westernised countries are:

1.   Eating too much and being overweight, which encourages oestrogen dominance and other important metabolic changes such as insulin resistance – a condition which means that the body no longer responds normally to insulin, and increases the risk of many gynae disorders, including polycystic ovary syndrome, fertility problems, fibroids, and breast cancer.

2.   Eating too little and becoming underweight. The hypothalamus responds to this by reducing the pituitary's production of ovary-stimulating hormones; this can stop ovulation and, perhaps, periods and can cause infertility.

3.   Eating an unhealthy diet. Taking in too much of certain nutrients and not enough of others encourages many gynae disorders.

alcohol

Many women enjoy drinking alcohol and, if done in moderation, this doesn't usually create problems. The advice on what constitutes moderate drinking and the size of a unit of alcohol, vary from country to country. In the UK, for example, moderate drinking (for women) means no more than two or three units a day – one unit being about 10ml (7.8g; 8g for convenience of calculation) of pure alcohol. But in the US, moderate drinking means no more than *one* unit a day – one unit being about 15ml (12g) of pure alcohol. Experts say, though, that drinking up to the limit each day is unwise and they recommend two to three alcohol-free days a week, and no binge drinking. They also suggest the limits should be less for under-18s and very slim women. As for pregnant women in the UK, for example, they are advised to drink no more than one or two UK units once or twice a week but in the US they are advised to abstain completely.

The problem is that not everyone agrees with these limits. Some experts point out that even moderate drinking raises the risk of certain gynae disorders and recommend at most 10ml of pure alcohol a day, 20ml only occasionally. Too much alcohol can reduce sex drive, raise stress-hormone levels, disturb menstrual cycles and harm unborn babies and, via breast milk, newborns. Continuing to drink too much over the months or years encourages surplus weight and can damage the liver, making it less able to break down surplus oestrogen. All this increases the likelihood of many gynae conditions, including period problems, polycystic ovaries, infertility and fibroids. Worryingly, any regular drinking encourages breast cancer; the more you drink the higher the risk. Six or more UK units (which is four or more US units, for example) a day encourage ovary cancer. An alcohol habit can damage arteries, reducing the health of the reproductive organs and sex-hormone glands. Finally, it raises the risk of osteoporosis by reducing the level of parathyroid hormone (needed to keep bones strong) and weakening the muscles (thereby reducing their strengthening 'pull' on bones).

The number of units in a drink depends on its volume and strength. The strength of a commercially produced alcohol beverage is indicated on its packaging as its AbV (alcohol by volume) – the number of millilitres of alcohol in every hundred millilitres. For example, 100ml of wine marked 8 per cent AbV contains 8ml of pure alcohol.

alchohol units in different countries

One unit in:

Ireland, UK	=	10ml	(8g)
Iceland	=	12ml	(9.5g)
Netherlands	=	12.5ml	(9.9g)
Australia, Italy, New Zealand, Spain	=	12.7ml	(10g)
Finland	=	13.9ml	(11g)
Denmark, France, Portugal, US	=	15ml	(12g)
Canada	=	17.1ml	(13.5g)
Hungary	=	21.5ml	(17g)
Japan	=	25ml	(19.75g)

As a rough guide, the AbV of beers is 2-7 per cent; wines 10-15 per cent; sherries and ports 20 per cent; and spirits and liqueurs 20-40 per cent. However, some varieties of each type of product have an AbV lower or higher than those in these ranges.

All this may seem rather complex, but it's important to be able to work out how much alcohol you're drinking, as so many women today drink too much. This is partly because, while they know how many units constitute 'moderate' drinking, they overestimate the size of a unit, thereby drinking more than they imagine.

making calculations

To calculate the number of millilitres of pure alcohol in a drink, multiply its AbV by its volume in millilitres, and divide the result by 100.

Then, to calculate the number of UK units in the drink, divide the number of millilitres of pure alcohol by the number of millilitres that constitutes a unit in your country.

For example, in the UK, if you have 125 millilitres (ml) of 12 per cent wine:

12 x 125 = 1500ml

1500 ÷ 100 = 15ml of pure alcohol

15ml ÷10ml (one UK unit) = 1.5 units

In fact, you get one UK unit in:

* 83ml (3fl oz) of 12 per cent wine

* 300ml (½ pint) of 3.5 per cent beer or cider (but the same volume of 5.5 per cent beer or cider contains 2 units)

* One measure (25ml) of spirits (Scotland has a bigger measure, giving 1.5 units,

And you get one US unit in:

* 100ml (3½fl oz) of 12 per cent wine

* 375ml (13fl oz) of 3.5 per cent beer or cider

* 1.5fl oz of spirits

Alcohol boosts the average woman's blood alcohol more than that of the average man for three reasons. Firstly, women are smaller and have a lower blood volume. Secondly, a woman's body contains relatively more fat and less water – so as fat absorbs less alcohol than does water, relatively more alcohol is available to enter the blood. And thirdly, a woman's stomach breaks down a smaller proportion of alcohol, as it produces 25 per cent less of an enzyme called dehydrogenase that detoxifies alcohol.

To keep your blood alcohol level relatively low, opt for spritzers, shandies, 5 per cent beers, or spirits topped up in a tall glass with plenty of mixer. Also, sip slowly; eat something, to slow the rate at which alcohol is absorbed into the blood and alternate alcoholic and soft drinks.

exercise

The main types of exercise include aerobic, strengthening and stretching (see Part three, page 263). All are important for gynae health, but particularly whole-body aerobic exercise and pelvic-floor exercises. Regular brisk aerobic exercise makes you sweat more and breathe faster. It also helps to keep every part of the body in good condition, including the heart, blood vessels, nerves, lungs, endocrine glands and 'women's bits'. It does this by boosting the blood supply, so that cells receive sufficient nutrients, hormones, immune factors and other vital substances to work well. In addition to this, it's a great help in maintaining a healthy weight and it also boosts endorphin levels, so lifting spirits and helping to counteract the many gynae conditions that can be fostered by anxiety, depression and stress. Too much exercise, on the other hand, makes the hypothalamus and pituitary decrease their production of ovary-stimulating hormones. This can prevent ovulation and make periods irregular – or even stop them altogether. It can also decrease immunity.

Pelvic-floor exercises (see Page 265) strengthen the 'hammock' of muscles that support the womb and bladder, helping to prevent or treat stress incontinence and prolapse.

breathing

While the average healthy woman, breathing normally, takes 13–17 breaths a minute, some get in the habit of breathing in an abnormally shallow and/or rapid way. Feeling stressed can make the chest muscles tense and encourage shallow breathing. Wearing a tight bra or belt can also encourage shallow breathing in a healthy woman, as can being pregnant or having indigestion. Excessively rapid breathing is known as 'hyperventilation' or 'over-breathing'. This means that a person exhales too much carbon dioxide which, in turn, makes their blood too alkaline, decreasing the oxygen available to cells. The cells in the hormone glands, reproductive system and other parts of the body therefore cannot function optimally, so almost any illness, gynaecological or otherwise, is more likely to occur. Hyperventilation often accompanies anxiety or stress (see page 45) but sometimes continues as a habit when life is easier. Very occasionally, hyperventilation is caused by an illness, such as diabetes or lung disease.

circulation

A good blood flow to and from hormone-producing glands and reproductive organs encourages them to be healthy and work well. The heart and blood vessels alter the blood flow in seconds in response to changes in the levels of nutrients, gases, hormones and neurotransmitters in the blood. The many lifestyle factors that encourage a healthy heart and arteries – and therefore good circulation – include:

- a healthy diet
- regular brisk aerobic exercise
- effective stress management

- being a non-smoker

- drinking alcohol only in moderation

- good relationships and laughter

micro-organisms

Billions of micro-organisms – including yeasts, moulds and other fungi, bacteria and protozoa – exist on the skin and in the body. Scientists call them 'flora' – for example, the bowel flora or vaginal flora. Their numbers and types depend on our health and diet and whether we've recently taken antibiotics, normally they help to keep us well. In the vagina, for example, they produce natural antibiotics and acids that ferment sugar in vaginal moisture to produce an acid that helps to prevent vaginal infection. In the bowel they encourage good digestion, promote regular bowel movements, counteract infections and they help to keep the body's oestrogen level healthy.

However, certain circumstances disturb their normal numbers and balance, causing 'dysbiosis' and this can affect gynae health. In the bowel, for example, it can result in constipation (which may raise the oestrogen level) or infection. In the vagina, dysbiosis can encourage a bacterial overgrowth called bacterial vaginosis or a candida infection (see Page 177).

light

Light stimulates the hypothalamus and pituitary to boost oestrogen and testosterone levels. It also encourages regular menstrual cycles and ovulation, so enhancing fertility. Bright light stimulates the pineal to make serotonin, which aids sexual functioning and combats stress. Darkness stimulates the pineal to make melatonin which influences sex drive, boosts immunity and is a powerful antioxidant – possibly even helping prevent certain cancers and other disorders. However, too much melatonin can make a woman less likely to ovulate, which encourages irregular periods and reduces fertility.

Lastly, sunlight enables the skin to produce vitamin D and is most women's main source of this vitamin. Having enough vitamin D helps to protect against osteoporosis and, because it helps to regulate normal cell division, may discourage certain cancers, including breast and colon cancer.

smoking

The more you smoke, the greater is the danger to your gynae and general health. Smoking over the years damages arteries, which reduces the blood flow to the reproductive organs and sex-hormone glands, rendering them less vital and perhaps making ovulation less regular and increasing the likelihood of infertilty and period problems. Smoking at any age encourages osteoporosis to develop earlier than it might otherwise have done. Smoking can bring the menopause forward by an average of two years because substances called polycyclic aromatic hydrocarbons in smoke make eggs die at a faster rate. Smoking after the menopause lowers the level of oestrogen, which may encourage hot flushes and other menopausal symptoms and makes a stroke or a heart attack more likely.

A woman who smokes has an increased risk of autoimmune diseases. Also, because smoking just one cigarette destroys 25mg of vitamin C, she may be short of this vitamin – which would encourage poor healing from any of the many disorders that involve infection or inflammation. She is more likely to have prematurely wrinkled skin, to develop rheumatoid arthritis, to become anxious or depressed and to get acne. Her baby is more likely to have a low birth weight, suffer from asthma or die from sudden infant death syndrome (cot or crib death). Finally, cancer-inducing (carcinogenic) substances from inhaled smoke encourage cancer of the cervix, vulva and breast (as well as certain non-gynae cancers, including lung cancer).

Many women who smoke do so to relieve stress. Indeed, in one survey in 1999, nearly one in two of the female smokers questioned said they felt they could not cope without smoking – mainly because it helped them deal with stress. Many of this group feared that if they gave up they would turn to food for comfort instead and then put on weight.

Help with stopping smoking is available as nicotine replacement therapy (from pharmacies), stop-smoking groups, counsellors, and a telephone helpline called Quitline (see the Helplist on page 000). The prescription-only 'stop-smoking' drug bupropion is another option but it isn't suitable for everyone and can have side effects, some of which may be severe.

pads, mini-pads, tampons and liners

In a recent survey, British women rated these second only to domestic electrical items as having had the most beneficial impact on women's lifestyles since 1945. Pads were first sold in the 1890s, disposable pads in 1921 and self-adhesive pads in the 1970s.

One less familiar type of 'sanitary protection' which has been around since the 1930s, is a rubber cup (see the Helplist, Page 315. This is inserted, folded, 1-2cm (⅖-⅘inch) into your vagina, where it unfolds and collects the menstrual flow. It holds up to 30ml (1fl oz) and needs emptying every four to six hours. Other types include small washable sponges, again inserted in the vagina and washable cloth pads.

Any form of sanitary protection alters the environment in the vagina and/or vulva. For example, wearing a tampon for too long, wearing one that's too absorbent or wearing one between periods, removes some of the vagina's protective moisture. It has also been linked with a very rare but potentially dangerous condition called toxic shock syndrome. (This is due to blood poisoning by toxins from a strain of *Staphylococcus aureus* bacteria present in the vagina in up to one in ten women and it shows up as a fever, restlessness, headache, a rash, and faintness.)

It is sensible to take precautions when using tampons. Use the lowest acceptable absorbency (choosing from 'junior', 'regular', 'super' and 'super plus'). Wash your hands before inserting one. Use tampons only during periods. Change your tampon every four hours during the day and insert a new one before bedtime and first thing in the morning – or, even better, use pads at night. Always remember to remove the last tampon of a period. If inserting a tampon feels uncomfortable, coat its tip with a

who uses what?

These figures, taken from a UK survey in September 2001, present percentages of menstruating women of different ages.

	Under-16s	16-18s	19-24s	25-34s	35+
Pads	96	90	62	62	71
Tampons	24	52	70	68	62
Liners	38	64	48	49	53

little lubricant (such as K-Y Jelly or another product suitable for use during sex). If it's uncomfortable in your vagina, you may not be pushing it in far enough, in which case the muscles around your vaginal opening may be tightening around it. If pain continues, or you have other symptoms, see your doctor in case you have an infection.

Wearing a pad, mini-pad or liner can make the vulva dry and, at worst, sore. It's wise to wear the least bulky one that will do the job, to change it more often if you get sore, and to wash your vulva twice a day during a period.

deodorants and anti-perspirants

A recent study found that at an unconscious level, a woman prefers the smell of the sweat of men whose MHC (major histocompatibility complex) genes are unlike her own. This may mean that detecting a man's natural scent – whether or not you're aware of it – is a good way of choosing a mate who isn't too similar to you genetically. In theory at any rate, this could reduce the chances of having a child with a genetic abnormality.

It is also possible that, at an unconscious level, the smell of a woman's sweat can influence men in making a biologically wise partner choice. Other research suggests that certain odoriferous substances in adult female sweat are particularly attractive to adult males; so the scent of a woman's sweat may be an important factor in attracting and keeping a mate. Indeed, many people think fresh sweat smells pleasant, some saying it can smell like freshly ground coffee. It's usually only as sweat spoils due to the action of bacteria that it starts to smell 'off' and people complain of 'BO'.

It's unlikely in this day and age that women in particular will give up using deodorants and antiperspirants. However, since most of these products are used only on the armpits, and pheromone-laden sweat continues to be produced in other areas (such as on the pubic area and the vulva, and around the nipples), it seems improbable that they will affect man-woman attraction in any significant way!

Certain deodorant sprays and wipes are marketed specifically for use on the vulva. However, some of their contents are irritating to some women so, from the 'gyn-ecology' point of view, they may be unwise.

sex and arousal

A positive and enjoyable sexual relationship helps a woman to feel happy, which has a beneficial effect on her gynae health by affecting the levels of many of her hormones and neurotransmitters.

In particular, sexual arousal, intercourse and orgasm alter the environment in the body and affect a woman's mindset in many valuable ways:

• Sexual arousal is often pleasurable, which boosts 'feel-good' hormones, may be an excellent stress-buster and can promote better bonding. Arousal also increases moisture production by the cervix and vagina, which protects the vagina from damage by friction from the penis. Lastly, arousal boosts the blood supply to the womb, vagina, ovaries, fallopian tubes and other pelvic structures, which helps to promote good gynae health.

• Physical activity during sex can be good exercise, especially if vigorous and not over too quickly! Ejaculated semen makes the normally acidic vagina relatively alkaline (this doesn't usually disrupt the balance of micro-organisms but a few women find that frequent sex without a condom encourages thrush).

• During orgasm, the hormone oxytocin makes the muscles of the womb, cervix and pelvic floor tense and relax in a series of rapid, powerful, rhythmical contractions. The associated pleasure and release of tension boosts our 'feel-good' factor, reduces stress-hormone levels, and aids sound sleep. Many women say an orgasm reduces period pain. Regular orgasms strengthen the pelvic floor, helping to prevent conditions such as stress incontinence and a prolapse. The contractions may help to dispel the pelvic 'heaviness' that's often blamed on pelvic congestion and may even help to prevent fibroids. However it's possible, though unproven, that women who frequently become aroused without having an orgasm are more likely to suffer from pelvic congestion.

non-human hormones

Some hormone-like substances from outside are nearly identical to certain of our own hormones. This allows them to become attached to matching cell receptors – so influencing the activity of these cells in the same way as do human hormones.

The Pill and HRT

The most common non-human hormones to which many of us are exposed are the oestrogens and progestogens ('progestins') in the Pill and HRT (hormone replacement therapy). Oestrogens, progestogens and other hormones are present in various gynae medications too. Progestogens are not identical to progesterone so, while they mimic some of its actions, they may also have some different ones.

The Pill and HRT can have a long-lasting influence on 'gyn-ecology', as some women take them for a very long time, so we'll consider their possible side effects here, on p.140 and also in Part Four. You'll find risk factors for serious side effects plus other information on the Pill and HRT in Part Four, along with details of other sex hormone medications.

HRT This contains oestrogen and progestogen or, if a woman no longer has her womb, oestrogen only and the doses are tiny compared with those in the Pill. Most of us manage the menopause without HRT – indeed, some of us feel better after our menopause than before. But others need a helping hand and some choose HRT. They may have menopausal hot flushes and night sweats, for example, that are so frequent as to be unacceptable; they may develop an uncomfortably dry vulva and vagina; and changes in the lining of their urine passage and bladder may encourage cystitis-like symptoms. Other women take HRT to reduce a high risk of osteoporosis or slow its development.

Many women have yet another agenda – they believe HRT to be a panacea that will keep them young, happy and sexy, and help to prevent age-related problems. However, while HRT certainly can have some benefits, in general this simply isn't so. Besides the fact that it can have side effects, HRT simply doesn't have the miraculous powers to reduce the progression of age-related disorders that some women hoped.

HRT can cause many relatively minor problems:

- monthly or three-monthly 'periods' from the 'sequential combined' type
- tender breasts, headaches, dizziness, cramp, depression, irritability, nausea, vomiting, dry eyes, itching, fluid retention, acne, brown skin patches on sun-exposed

does HRT help to prevent?

Flushes and sweats	Yes
Osteoporosis	Yes
Dry or sore vulva and vagina	Yes
Bowel cancer	Yes
Lines and wrinkles	Yes (removes fine lines by encouraging fluid retention and so thickening the skin)
Dry vagina and vulva	Yes
Cystitis due to lack of oestrogen in the lining of the bladder and urethra (urine passage from the bladder to the vulva)	Yes
Sleep problems, fatigue and depression	Not clear, partly because they so often have other causes
Low sex drive and responsiveness	Possibly
Memory loss	Possibly
Dental problems	Possibly
Osteoarthritis	Possibly
Leg ulcers and pressure sores	Possibly
Alzheimer's disease	Possibly (we'll know more when a long-term trial ends in 2011)
Heart disease	No
Strokes	No

skin and irregular vaginal 'spotting' of blood occur in one in six women but tend to go within a few months

• a rash and itching from skin patch adhesive

• an increase in vaginal moisture that's enough to warrant wearing a mini-pad, pad or tampon, from oestrogen-only HRT

• irritation, itching, infection, and ulceration from oestrogen-containing products for the vagina or vulva

More seriously, HRT can:

• trigger asthma and jaundice, raise blood pressure, encourage varicose veins, suppress immunity, and make gallstones more than three times as likely (if taken for longer than two years)

• raise the risk of breast cancer; the increase is relatively small (if 10,000 women took long term combined HRT for a year, eight more than expected would get breast cancer), but the longer you're on HRT, the greater the risk becomes. The increased risk disappears once you've been off it for five years. Also, several studies suggest that breast cancer in women on HRT is less likely to be fatal, partly because they tend to have more regular mammograms and other breast checks, and partly because it tends to be a less aggressive sort of cancer

• encourage ovary, liver and skin cancer

• increase the risk of womb cancer, in the case of long-term sequential HRT

• raise the risk – according to a recent large US study – of heart attacks, strokes and potentially dangerous blood clots. However, each individual's risk each year is fairly small. For example, if 10,000 women took long term combined HRT for a year, seven more than expected would suffer from a heart attack, eight a stroke and 18 a blood clot.

Plant oestrogens (phyto-oestrogens)

Certain foods (see page 260) contain plant oestrogens that are similar enough to our own oestrogens to have some oestrogenic activity in our body, so they can help to prevent or treat certain gynae conditions. They do this by becoming attached to oestrogen receptors in many parts of the body, including the breasts, womb, ovaries, bladder, bone, brain and thymus. Alpha-receptors are found mostly in breast and womb cells and beta-receptors mostly in brain (especially pituitary, hypothalamus, and learning and memory centres), bone, ovary, heart, blood vessel, lung, kidney and bladder cells. Plant oestrogens have a higher affinity for beta-receptors.

If plant oestrogens become attached to receptors when the levels of a woman's own, more powerful oestrogens are high, they block the receptors so that her own oestrogens can't influence cell behaviour. There is reason to believe that the overall effect of this in a pre-menopausal woman could be a decrease in the oestrogenic activity in her body, which might help to prevent problems associated with an oestrogen-dominant hormone imbalance (see page 89). However, if the levels of her own oestrogens are low, as after the menopause for example, plant oestrogens can increase the oestrogenic activity in her body.

It's possible that plant oestrogens may also help to prevent problems arising from xeno-oestrogens (see below).

Xeno-oestrogens ('foreign' oestrogens)

These include synthetic substances that can behave like weak oestrogens, such as nonylphenol, which can enter food from soft plastic or polystyrene food packaging; bisphenyl A, which can contaminate food from the lacquer coating the inside of some cans and certain solvents and pesticides. Dioxins can also have oestrogenic activity. These organochlorine substances are widespread environmental contaminants, present in many foods and derived from such things as paper and pesticide manufacture and the burning – in municipal incinerators and elsewhere – of plastics, coal, solvents, wood treated with preservatives, and the stubble of crops treated with pesticides.

contraception

If 100 sexually active women use no contraception for a year, 80 to 90 will get pregnant. So the effectiveness of each method in preventing pregnancy is quoted as the number of women in every 100 who don't get pregnant using that method according to instructions. However, besides preventing pregnancy contraception can influence gynae health in many other ways.

Condoms, diaphragms and caps

Condoms (both 'male' and the vastly less popular 'female') are the only contraceptive methods to give considerable protection against sexually transmitted infections. Using a spermicidal foam, gel, or cream is essential if you use a diaphragm or a cap, and wise if you use a condom (in case it breaks). Spermicidal products rarely cause problems, though some women are sensitive to them and may develop an itchy vulva, for example. Condoms, diaphragms and

how well contraceptive methods work

Method	Effective in (per 100 women per year)
Male condoms	98
Female condoms	95
Combined Pill	Over 99
Progestogen-only Pill	99
Diaphragm or cap	92-96
Intrauterine device (coil)	Over 99
Intrauterine system	Over 99
Injections	Over 99
Implants	Over 99
Natural family planning	Up to 98
Lactational amenorrhoea method	See page 44
Emergency contraception	Can prevent 7 in 8 pregnancies
Sterilisation	1 in 200 female sterilisations fails in a lifetime
	1 in 2000 male sterilisations fails after 2 clear tests

caps can all reduce a woman's pleasure from sex. Anyone wanting protection against sexually transmitted infections along with a high level of protection against pregnancy should use both a condom and a hormonal method such as the Pill.

Hormonal contraception

The Pill, hormone-releasing coils, skin patches, implants and injections and emergency contraception all alter the environment in a woman's body by changing her hormone balance.

The Pill This either prevents a fertilised egg from becoming attached to the womb lining, or prevents ovulation. It eases some period problems, and makes ovary and womb cancer less likely. Indeed, research suggests that being on the Pill for five years can halve the risk of ovary cancer, because it suppresses ovary-stimulating hormones; this could be useful for women in families where this cancer has occurred. Research also suggests that being on the Pill halves the risk of womb cancer (probably because of its progestogen content).

However, the Pill has many possible side effects, though most are uncommon, and the potentially serious ones are rare:

The combined (oestrogen plus progestogen) Pill can cause:

•   nausea, constipation, gallstones, weight gain, fluid retention, headache, cramp, migraine, tender breasts, vaginal discharge, reduced sex drive, depression, erosion of the cervix, and cystitis

•   high blood pressure

•   inflamed veins

•   a tendency for the blood to clot. This can cause a blood clot in a leg vein (deep vein thrombosis), which can be fatal if a piece breaks off and travels to the lungs (pulmonary embolism). It can also cause a stroke due to a blood clot in a brain artery or a heart attack due to a blood clot in a coronary artery. These blood clotting problems are more likely in women who smoke and the risk rises with age. Around 6 per cent of women have a genetic defect that makes their blood more likely to clot on the Pill, and one day it may be possible to test for this so that they can choose other forms of contraception

•   breast cancer, though the increase in risk is only very slight. In every thousand women on the Pill, one extra will get this cancer compared with the same number not on the Pill; this increased risk disappears ten years after stopping the Pill and is almost certainly related to the Pill's oestrogen. However, the Pill may not actually 'cause' this extra risk; it's perhaps more likely either that it encourages existing isolated cancer cells (which might otherwise be destroyed by a woman's immune system) to multiply, so that breast cancer appears sooner or that it's picked up earlier because women on the Pill tend to see their doctor more often

•   While a close family history of breast cancer raises your own breast cancer risk, researchers don't believe that taking the Pill increases this risk further

• malignant melanoma (a potentially dangerous skin cancer). In one study, women on the Pill had twice the risk of contracting this cancer and those who took it for over ten years had a threefold risk. But this applied only if a woman already had a raised risk due to having red or blonde hair, melanoma in the family or previous sunburn. The raised risk is almost certainly related to the Pill's oestrogen; however, a woman's risk fell to normal within two years of stopping the Pill. This suggests that oestrogen doesn't cause cancer (if it did, the risk would be high for many years) but that it encourages existing isolated cancer cells – which might otherwise be destroyed by the immune system – to multiply.

The progestogen-only ('mini') Pill can cause:

• disrupted periods, bleeding between periods, nausea, headaches, depression, tender breasts, bloating, and weight gain

The Pill in general may:

• prevent the normal increase in sensitivity to smell around ovulation (research suggests this may affect partner choice by altering a woman's response to male pheromones)

• interact with certain other drugs so that it no longer provides effective contraception. These drugs include certain antibiotics and many older epilepsy drugs (including phenytoin, carbamazepine, phenobarbitone, primidone and topirimate). The concern with epilepsy drugs and the Pill isn't just that a woman may become pregnant when she doesn't want to but that, if she does become pregnant, the epilepsy drugs may damage her unborn baby before she knows she is expecting. The good news is that newer drugs (such as sodium valproate, lamotrigine and vigabatrin) have no effect on the Pill.

Delaying a period:

You can use the Pill to delay your next period if its timing would be inconvenient. With most brands this means not taking the packet's last seven inactive or 'dummy' pills (the ones that allow a 'period' or, more accurately, a 'breakthrough bleed') but starting a new packet at once. Check with your doctor, though, as it's different with some brands. (If you aren't on the Pill, and want to delay a period, ask your doctor to consider prescribing a progestogen

– such as norethisterone, 5mg three times a day – to take from three days before you expect your period until three days before it's acceptable to have one).

The hormone-releasing intra-uterine system This is a fine tube, inserted via the vagina and cervix into the womb, which prevents pregnancy by slowly releasing a progestogen. The amount is so small (equivalent to two progestogen-only Pills a week) that side effects (such as acne, headaches, bloating, nausea, and tender breasts) are very unlikely. However, as it's a bit wider than a coil, a local anaesthetic may be necessary to facilitate its insertion. Occasional light bleeding ('spotting') between periods is common for three months. It can be left in for five years. However, in around one in five women it either comes out spontaneously during the first year, or causes bleeding between periods bad enough to warrant removal.

Hormone implants and injections These contain progestogens, which can cause nausea, tender breasts and headaches. In some places (such as Latin America) contraceptive injections can also contain oestrogen.

Emergency contraception (morning-after pill) This contains a high dose of a progestogen called levonorgestrel. This either prevents ovulation, or prevents a fertilised egg from implanting in the womb lining. It works in up to four in five women if taken within 72 hours of unprotected sex, though taking it within 12 hours makes it more effective. Having a coil (see below) inserted within five days of unprotected sex is even more effective.

Intra-uterine contraceptive device (IUCD, IUD, or 'coil')

A doctor inserts this plastic and copper device into the womb; very occasionally the cervix must be dilated first. The coil prevents fertilisation and/or a fertilised egg from implanting in the womb lining.

If there's any chance that you could have a sexually transmitted infection, inserting the coil could encourage womb infection and pelvic inflammatory disease. This is a particular problem with chlamydia. So your doctor will either arrange a chlamydia test before inserting a coil or, if infection is likely, give you a dose of antibiotics. A coil can trigger painful, heavy or irregular periods and back pain. Having a coil inserted within five days of unprotected sex is a 100 per cent successful method of 'emergency contraception'.

Sterilisation

Having the fallopian tubes cut, tied, sealed or clipped during a laparoscopy is a popular and effective contraceptive method. It usually involves a general anaesthetic and there may be a short-term stomachache afterwards.

Ovulation can still occur after sterilisation, but instead of entering a fallopian tube the egg simply disappears and is absorbed without trace.

Occasionally sterilisation can damage tiny blood vessels that supply the ovaries and make one or both ovaries unable to ovulate, causing irregular and, perhaps, lighter periods. It's unlikely to be reversible.

Natural family planning

The following methods can be very effective – but only if you know exactly how to use them.

Avoiding sex when fertile One way of doing this is to learn to detect the changes in vaginal moisture, cervix, and body temperature associated with the fertile time of the month. Another is by using urine dipsticks and an electronic ovulation monitor (see the Helplist, page 315) to detect the changes in the urine levels of hormones associated with the fertile time. This has no side effects but can be frustrating in that many women feel at their most sexy during the fertile time of the month, so some couples decide to use a condom, or a diaphragm plus spermicide, then.

Lactational amenorrhoea method (LAM) A breastfeeding woman who feeds her baby frequently and regularly and whose baby has unlimited sucking time and no dummy, can hope to suppress ovulation for over a year after the baby's birth. Indeed, in the average woman who has breastfed exclusively and on an unrestricted basis for six to eight months, then has introduced solids but continued to breastfeed frequently, ovulation doesn't return until her baby is 15-27 months old. The very earliest it may happen is in the tenth week and the woman has only a one-in-20 chance of ovulating before the eighteenth week. If the mother of a baby under six months has not yet had her first period and gives at least six (preferably more) feeds, well spaced throughout the day and night, LAM gives a better than 98 per cent chance of avoiding pregnancy. The average time before periods return in a woman breastfeeding this way is over 14 months.

LAM is most effective when used in conjunction with fertility awareness methods (see above). This is because some woman ovulate for the first time two weeks before their first period. Also, any disruption to frequent, regular breastfeeding (or expression of milk – which has a similar effect on a woman's ovary-stimulating hormones) may trigger ovulation. So a woman needs to be on the alert for ovulation and either avoid sex or use a condom or a diaphragm and spermicide when natural family planning techniques indicate that she is fertile. The drawback is that ovulation isn't always as easy to detect in a breastfeeding woman as it is in a non-breastfeeding one so, while LAM is the world's single most important method of spacing babies, it isn't the most reliable.

emotions, stress, relaxation and laughter

These have a profound influence on gynae health because of their close links with hormone and neurotransmitter levels. For example, feeling joyful raises the levels of 'feel-good' hormones and, conversely, it can also result from a rise in the levels of 'feel-good' hormones – due, for example, to half an hour's brisk exercise.

Similarly, feeling stressed can raise the levels of stress hormones such as adrenaline and stress can also come about as a result of a rise in these levels – due, for example, to smoking. In particular, stress can alter the levels of ovary-stimulating hormones causing heavy periods and, perhaps, preventing periods and ovulation.

relationships

The way in which we relate to others alters hormone and neurotransmitter levels and balances. So the quality of relationships – particularly close ones – can have an enormously powerful effect on general and gynae health. The good news is that there are many practical and proven tools we can use to improve our relationships, among them being skills for effective listening, stress-management, assertiveness training, conflict-resolution and encouragement (see Part Three, page 253–291).

sexual abuse and female 'circumcision'

Needless to say, these have far-reaching effects on gynae health. Conscious and unconscious memories of sexual abuse can affect a woman's sexuality, self-esteem and stress-management skills. Her relationships with men and with doctors (including gynaecologists and obstetricians), and her parenting skills may also suffer. Indeed, such experiences can haunt her throughout her life until such time as she can get help or find ways of managing her response to them.

As for female 'circumcision', 2 million girls (mostly from 28 African countries, including Sudan, Somalia, Djibouti and Ethiopia) are forced to undergo this unnecessary and mutilating genital operation. At worst, the operator (not usually a doctor) cuts off the girl's clitoris and inner labia, then sews up the outer labia, leaving a tiny hole for the menstrual flow, urine, sex and childbirth. One aim is to enhance fidelity to a future partner by destroying an important source of sexual pleasure. However, the operation also carries a high risk of infection and bleeding, encourages urine infections and can lead to enormous difficulty in giving birth. Thankfully the World Health Organisation is raising awareness so that girls have the knowledge, confidence and support to refuse circumcision and older women realise they don't have to impose this archaic custom on their daughters.

good gynae health for life

Although this may depend partly on our genes, we can encourage it by taking on board five key lifestyle strategies and checking we know how to protect our gynae health during each stage of life.

genes

Our genes encourage certain gynae conditions and discourage others. Until recently there has been little we could do about this other than to have more frequent screening tests if necessary (for example, if a close female relative has an illness with a strong genetic influence such as oestrogen-sensitive breast cancer). However, over the last few decades it has become increasingly obvious that environmental factors can encourage or prevent the action of certain genes. This puts our genetic blueprint under our personal control in a way that was previously believed to be impossible.

Scientists are working on tests for many genetically influenced conditions and are unravelling ways in which a woman can change certain factors in her environment so as to reduce her risk of particular gynae conditions. For example, if oestrogen-sensitive breast cancer runs in her family, she could try to lower her risk by reducing her alcohol intake and avoiding exposure to oestrogens such as those in HRT.

Five key physical lifestyle strategies

The five key physical lifestyle strategies that encourage good health in general, and good gynae health in particular, at any age or stage in life are:

• eating a healthy diet

• taking regular exercise

• not smoking

• managing stress effectively

• drinking alcohol only in moderation.

(For more detailed information, see pages 255,263,32,266,27.)

gynae health for baby and child

We tend not to think of gynae health as being relevant to children, but there are several concerns.

Caring for a baby girl's breasts and vulva

Ignore any swelling of your newborn baby daughter's breasts as it will soon go. Wash her vulva gently each day with plenty of water and a little soap or cleanser if necessary. If her vulva or bottom becomes at all sore, leave the nappy off as much as possible so that air and light can aid healing. Smooth barrier cream over her vulva and around her bottom to help prevent irritation from a wet or soiled nappy.

Promoting good self-esteem and healthy attitudes

The attitudes, moral values and self-esteem that your daughter accumulates in her early years, together with the listening, assertion and conflict-resolution skills she learns, will shape her views and behaviours and strongly influence the way in which she'll manage her gynae health in years to come. Most of her attitudes and moral values come from observing you, the rest of her family and other carers, her peer group, the characters in soaps and other TV programmes and her schoolteachers and religious educators. Help your daughter to grow up without embarrassment or shame about her body by not being self-conscious about your own nudity and by answering questions about genitals and sex in a matter-of-fact and age-appropriate way. Make sure she knows about periods well before her first one is likely to occur – which could be when she's as young as nine (see page 19) and take time to discuss relationships and sex whenever these subjects arise. Remember, though, that actions speak louder than words, so the way in which you handle your own relationships and learn from mistakes is particularly important.

gynae health in the teenage years

Important issues with gynae implications for teens include periods, relationships and sex, contraception, sexually transmitted diseases, and screening tests for chlamydia infection and cervix cancer.

Periods

Some girls have regular periods from the start, while in others periods are irregular for some months or even years. Heavy periods are a problem for some girls until their menstrual cycles are well established. In contrast, regular ovulation and periods can encourage period pain. Period problems can be frustrating, especially if they interfere with activities and make it difficult to plan. Try not to worry because regular menstrual hormone cycles and ovulation are relatively easily disrupted in younger teenagers yet the odds of cycles settling down are extremely strong.

Relationships and sex

The pressures on a teenage girl today to have sex are high. They come from the media, your peer group and the opposite sex, as well as from your own biologically determined interest in sex. Yet the traditional brakes on early sex – such as religious teaching and disapproval from parents and society in general – are often much less effective than they were a couple of generations ago. This explains why, according to one UK survey for example, one girl in three has had sex before the age of 16.

Early sex can be a problem for several reasons. For one thing, seven in 10 girls in the above UK survey who had sex before they were 16 regretted it and one in five said they had been forced into it. For another, you risk sexually transmitted infection and unplanned and, perhaps, unwanted pregnancy. Unplanned pregnancy is often associated with single motherhood and single mothers are more likely than married or otherwise partnered ones to be lonely and financially poor. The babies of teen mothers

– especially single ones – are more likely to die in infancy (which sounds dreadful but is a stark fact), to grow up without their father being around, to be sexually abused, to have problems with drink and drugs and to become single teen mothers themselves.

Postponing sex can foster self-respect and demonstrate that you value a boy as a person rather than a sex object. It can also show that you believe sex is too important at emotional and spiritual levels to be squandered in a casual relationship. However, you need the right skills to be able to say 'no' without feeling prudish or 'un-cool' or hurting a boy's feelings. Some schools run workshops that provide the opportunity to practise these skills. Not having sex until you are married (or in some other loving, committed, long-term partnership) makes a valued relationship much more likely to last. Whether or not a girl consciously plans on having early sex, a high sex drive, adventurousness, curiosity and a host of unconscious issues may drive her to it. So every girl needs to know how to protect herself from pregnancy and how to prevent and detect sexually transmitted disease.

Contraception

However sophisticated your knowledge, it's worth reminding yourself of two things:

- never to believe that you won't get pregnant because it's 'the wrong time of the month', since with 'unprotected' sex (sex without contraception) it's possible to get pregnant at any time of the menstrual cycle

- never to trust the 'withdrawal method', in which the boy removes his penis from your vagina after he has ejaculated ('come'), since a few drops containing sperm can leave the penis some time before ejaculation.

(See pages 39-45 for reliable methods of contraception.)

Sexually transmitted infection

Again, however sophisticated your knowledge, the following points are worth remembering:

- Unless you and your partner have only ever had sex with each other, it's important to protect yourselves against infection (see 'Safer sex', page 199)

- The Pill provides no protection against infection – for this your partner needs to use a condom.

• Using a spermicidal foam, gel or cream with a condom or diaphragm offers no additional protection against sexually transmitted infection.

It's wise to get medical help if there is the slightest suspicion that you have caught an infection – chlamydia infection, for example, is not only very common but can be symptom-free for years.

Screening

Some teens need screening tests for chlamydia infection and cervix cancer.

For chlamydia infection

Some doctors recommend regular chlamydia screening for every sexually active girl.

• **Why?** Because although chlamydia infection may not cause any obvious symptoms, it's common and can lead to infertility.

• **How?** A doctor or nurse takes a sample of the moisture from your upper vagina and sends it to a laboratory for tests.

• **How often?** Every six months.

For cervix cancer

While routine cervical (Pap) smears are recommended in the USA at least every three years from the onset of sexual activity, and in Australia every two years starting at age 18 (or one or two years after becoming sexually active), they are not recommended for teens in the UK. This is because normal developmental changes can make a smear wrongly appear 'abnormal', and also because if there are abnormal cells, they are likely to be only very mildly abnormal and it's considered safe to wait for routine screening from 20 onwards to pick them up.

gynae health in the 20s, 30s and 40s

Important gynae concerns to bear in mind at this stage include contraception, preventing and detecting sexually transmitted diseases, breast awareness and screening.

Contraception

Many women choose the Pill, but unless you and your partner are both virgins, or have been faithful for many months and are free from sexually transmitted infections, it's wise to use a condom as well, to protect against such infections.

Before starting the Pill remember the following:

• You will need a medical check.

• The choice of brand should suit your age, reproductive stage, and medical history. Combined oral contraceptive Pills (with oestrogen and progestogen) contain 20-50 micrograms of oestrogen – those with the relatively lower level are less likely to have oestrogenic side effects but carry a very slightly higher risk of pregnancy.

• Some types result in no periods for months at a time and you may have scanty or irregular periods, especially early on.

• You should see a doctor urgently if you experience leg pain or swelling, chest pain, breathlessness, a severe headache or weakness in one side of your body,

when to see a doctor

You

You should see a doctor if you have:

• an abnormal vaginal discharge

• a sore vulva or vagina

• an itchy vulva

• unexplained low abdominal pain

• bleeding between periods or after sex

• an unexplained fever

• genital blisters or ulcers

• pain or discomfort during sex

• pain on passing urine

Your partner

Your partner should see a doctor if he has:

• a discharge from his penis

• pain on passing urine

• a rash or other skin changes on his genitals

or if you cough up blood-stained mucus, as you may have a potentially dangerous blood clot.

• If you are late taking a Pill (over 12 hours for the combined Pill, or three for the progestogen-only Pill), if you have severe vomiting or diarrhoea or if you take antibiotics, you need to be sure of your continued protection against pregnancy. Either read the instructions in the Pill pack, or ask your doctor.

(see also pages 39-45 for other methods of contraception.)

Preventing sexually transmitted diseases

Both casual sex and repeated short-lived faithful relationships readily spread sexually transmitted infections. An infection can, however, be 'silent' with no obvious symptoms so, unless you and your new partner are absolutely sure that you are infection-free and have had no other partner in the last few months, use condoms for several months, even if you are on the Pill.

Breast awareness

Be aware of how your breasts are from day to day and month to month, so that you can report anything unusual or unexpected to your doctor right away. This includes changes in colour, texture, shape and the direction in which the nipples point, as well as lumps that continue after a period. The earlier breast cancer is detected and treated the better the outcome.

Ongoing breast awareness (see page 60) is better than 'formal' monthly breast checks. (When the Canadian Task Force on Preventive Health Care reviewed the research, they concluded that formal monthly breast checks by 40-69-year-old women did not reduce their risk of fatal breast cancer; there isn't enough evidence to say for sure whether formal checks are wise in other age groups.)

Screening

In their 20s, 30s or 40s, only a few women need routine mammograms, all need routine smears and some need regular chlamydia tests.

For breast cancer

In the US, routine mammograms are recommended every one to two years, in Australia they are not recommended (but are available on request every two years) and in the UK experts currently don't believe there is enough evidence to recommend routine mammograms in women under 50. Women who have had breast or ovary cance, or who have a close relative (mother, sister or daughter) with such cancers, may be advised to start having routine mammograms earlier.

For cervix cancer

Routine cervical (Pap) smears are recommended in the USA every year in women aged 20-64, in Australia every two years (perhaps from 18, see above) and in the UK every three to five years from 20-64. Women who have cervical cell abnormalities need more frequent smears.

For chlamydia infection

Regular tests are wise for any sexually active woman unless she is having sex only with one faithful partner. Depending on your sexual history, your doctor may recommend a test as often as every six to twelve months.

gynae health in pregnancy and when breastfeeding

When you are pregnant you can ensure that your unborn baby's general (and gynae if it's a girl) health get off to a good start by getting good obstetric care yourself and checking that your own lifestyle won't harm her. A good diet encourages healthy growth and development in the baby and helps prevent a premature delivery. It may also reduce the baby's future risk of diabetes and arterial disease (leading, perhaps, to high blood pressure, heart disease and 'brain attacks' (strokes)). Diabetes, for example, can reduce a woman's fertility and encourage miscarriage and both diabetes and heart disease can reduce the circulation to any part of the body including a woman's reproductive organs – and so make them function less well than before.

Keeping active helps to maintain healthy blood vessels, including those in the placenta), helps prevent you from getting overly fat (which encourages miscarriage) and guards against high blood pressure and diabetes (which can be hazardous for an unborn baby).

Twenty to 30 minutes of bright outdoor daylight a day provides vitamin D, which aids the absorption from food of the calcium that's needed to keep your bones strong during pregnancy.

Being a non-smoker helps your unborn baby to grow and develop well and, most importantly, have a healthy birth weight. The nicotine and other toxic chemicals your baby receives from your blood if you smoke reduce her blood supply so encouraging a low birth weight. This raises the risk of several problems after birth including breathing difficulties and later life problems, such as high blood pressure, diabetes and heart disease.

It's wise to breastfeed exclusively, day and night, for six months if you can and to carry on until your baby is at least a year old. You may meet challenges – such as fearing you don't have enough milk – but you can almost certainly overcome them, with help, if necessary, from a professional health adviser, a trained breastfeeding counsellor or a book such as my *Breast is Best*.

There are many reasons why mother's milk is the best food for babies. It reduces the risk of many health problems in childhood or later life, including infections, allergies, type-1 diabetes (the sort that comes on suddenly in childhood) and heart disease. Breastfeeding also has benefits for you. For example, oxytocin – which enables the breasts to release milk – also causes womb contractions that speed the return of the womb and cervix to their pre-pregnant state. Also, long term breastfeeding helps to prevent pre-menopausal breast cancer, and, perhaps, womb cancer.

gynae health around the menopause and later

Contraception remains an important gynae concern around the menopause and screening is particularly important from the age of 50 onwards.

Contraception

Although fertility is reduced around the menopause, conception is still possible, so it's wise to continue using contraception for two years after your last period if this was before the age of 50, and one year if it was after. If you've been using condoms, spermicidal foam alone is considered a good enough contraceptive once you are 50.

The Pill

If you stay on this you'll have regular Pill-induced bleeds after the menopause and the oestrogen in a 'combined' Pill will prevent menopausal flushes and sweats (though the progestogen-only Pill won't). This means that you won't know when you've had your menopause. You now have three choices:

• Stop the combined Pill every year after 50 and use condoms or a diaphragm instead. Then either wait to see if your periods return or, two weeks after stopping the Pill, have a blood test to measure your levels of follicle stimulating hormone (FSH) and oestradiol (a type of oestrogen) or a saliva test for oestrogen and progesterone levels. Around the menopause, FSH tends to rise and oestrogen to fall. A relatively high FSH level (over 20 international units per litre) would suggest that you've had your menopause, meaning it will be safe to stop using contraception a year from now. (However, this isn't completely reliable, as the FSH level fluctuates considerably around the menopause and can be low one day and high the next.)

• Change to – or stay on – the progestogen-only Pill. This doesn't interfere with the FSH/oestradiol test, so you can have the test done while continuing to take this Pill.

• Stop the combined Pill when you are 54, as your periods are highly likely to have stopped by then, though you'll need to use condoms or a diaphragm for a further year to be sure. The only problem here is that any health risks from taking the Pill after the age of 50 are unknown.

Other contraception

If you have a progestogen-releasing intrauterine device and have unacceptable menopausal flushes and sweats, ask your doctor about using oestrogen tablets or patches or an oestrogen gel.

Contraception on HRT

Some women wonder whether taking HRT during and after the menopause will protect them from conceiving. The answer is it won't, because its oestrogen dose isn't high enough to prevent ovulation.

If you take HRT while still having periods it can be a challenge to recognise your menopause and so to know when to stop contraception. There are three ways of managing this:

• If you're 51 (the average age for the menopause) or older, try – preferably after discussion with your doctor – coming off HRT, though reduce it gradually, over three months, as stopping suddenly provokes flushes and sweats. When you've been off it for six weeks ask your doctor for a blood test to check your level of follicle stimulating hormone (FSH – see 'The Pill', above). If this is relatively high it suggests you've had your menopause and it will be safe to stop using contraception a year from now.

• If you are 51 or more, you could come off HRT slowly now, and continue using a barrier contraceptive (condom or diaphragm) until you've been free from periods for a year.

• You could continue with HRT and contraception until 55, then come off HRT slowly and stop contraception at the same time, as conception is extremely unlikely.

Screening tests after 50

Regular screening tests for cancer of the cervix and of the breast is advisable. Some doctors also recommend an ultrasound scan of the ovaries every few years, especially if there is ovary or breast cancer in your family. Breast cancer becomes increasingly common with age, so continue to be 'breast aware' (see page 60) and report any concerns to your doctor.

For breast cancer

In the US routine mammograms are recommended every one to two years up to the age of 74, in Australia every two years up to the age of 69 (but they are available on request to 79) and in the UK every three years up to the age of 64 (but they are available on request for older women, and will be offered routinely to the age of 70 by 2004).

Many experts believe that there isn't enough evidence to back routine mammograms for women over the age of 70.

For cervix cancer

Routine cervical (Pap) smears are recommended for women in the USA every year until they are 64, in Australia every two years until they are 70, and in the UK every three to five years again until they are 64.

Women who have cervical cell abnormalities need more frequent smears.

part two / gynae concerns and conditions

In this section you will find information on common gynae disorders arranged in sections according to where the main symptoms are located. For each disorder there are details of symptoms, causes and triggers. There are guidelines on how to prevent or treat it yourself and when to see the doctor, as well as a brief description of any medical tests or investigations the doctor may do and possible medical treatments. Finally, there's a simple, at-a-glance, treatment plan at the end of each entry.

I have chosen home remedies and therapies either because there is good scientific evidence that they work or because common sense dictates that this is likely and they won't do any harm. I have not included homeopathic treatments because, although experience often suggests they can help, there isn't enough space here to do them justice and, although the idea of their gentleness and, perhaps, specificity is very attractive, there is very little scientific evidence indeed to support their use.

At the end of the entry for each symptom, you'll find a list of its possible gynae or gynae-related causes, in order of likelihood; for possible gynae or gynae-related causes of more general symptoms, such as backache, consult the end of Part Two (pages 223-252). Note that non-gynae or non-gynae-related causes are not included in these 'symptom sorter' lists.

Further details of 'natural' cures can be found in Part Three (see pages 253-291), and there is more information on medical tests, investigations and treatments in Part Four (pages 293-312).

breasts

Our breasts work hard throughout our reproductive life, changing in shape, density and structure with fluctuations in hormone levels. And all our adult life they are important as sources of sexual pleasure and symbols of femininity. In this section we'll look at breast lumps, skin changes, swelling, pain and size as well as nipple itching and discharge, and breast cancer.

breast lump(s)

General lumpiness

One in three women sometimes has lumpy breasts, especially in the week or two before her period. Tenderness and pain may also occur. The lumps are usually similar in size and consistency and most likely to occur in each breast's upper outer quadrant ('quarter'). This is known as 'benign breast changes' or diffuse nodularity. Older names include benign breast disease, fibroadenosis, fibrocystic disease and chronic cystic mastitis. A large lump is most likely to be a cyst (a tough fluid-filled 'bag'), though a fibroadenoma (a rubbery growth of fibrous and glandular tissue) is fairly common. This sort of lumpiness may result from oestrogen – indicating an oestrogen-dominant hormone imbalance (see page 89) – or from sensitivity of milk-gland cells to oestrogen, progesterone or prolactin or to changing levels of these and other sex hormones. Some women develop lumpiness when they take HRT. The lumps are benign, but women with benign lumps can develop breast cancer and surveys suggest that they have one and a half times the average woman's risk. Researchers don't yet know whether taking the Pill encourages these lumps.

An unusual or unexpected lump

If your breasts aren't usually lumpy or if you are post-menopausal, a lump is most likely to be a fibroadenoma or cyst. Another possibility is an area of 'reactive' hardening (fibrosis) at the base of the breast (perhaps due to pressure from a badly fitting bra) or a swollen milk duct – perhaps due to 'duct ectasia',

59

(see page 66) or, in a breastfeeding woman, a blocked milk duct. A lump might also be a fatty growth (lipoma), a wart-like growth (papilloma) in a milk duct or a cancer – which is why you should never ignore a new lump. The good news is that nine out of 10 unusual or unexpected lumps are benign.

what to do yourself

Breast awareness – Be aware of how your breasts feel and look from day to day. This way you get to know what's normal for you and are more likely to recognise any unusual lump or other breast or nipple changes early on (see Breast cancer, page 73) that need to be checked for cancer. Note the dates of your periods and the daily state of the lumpiness, to see if it changes with your menstrual cycle and is therefore hormone-sensitive.

Right-size bra – Tight bras can make the breasts congested by obstructing the flow in blood and lymph vessels. The resulting pressure of surplus tissue fluid around the cells might encourage breast tissue to defend itself by forming lumps.

Healthy weight maintenance – to make it easier to spot significant breast changes early.

Also, for hormone-sensitive lumps:

Discourage oestrogen dominance (page 89).

Cut down on coffee, tea, cola, cocoa and chocolate – in the week or so before a period, as their caffeine or other methylxanthines can aggravate lumpiness. If you notice you crave chocolate before a period, try cutting it out for a couple of months just in case it's encouraging lumpiness.

symptom sorter

Gynae or gynae-related causes of breast lump(s)

● ● ● **Most likely** – benign breast changes, reactive hardening, blocked milk duct (when breastfeeding), single fibroadenoma or cyst, milk-duct papilloma

● ● **Less likely** – duct ectasia

● **Possible** – lipoma, breast cancer

Exercise – Both whole-body aerobic exercise and arm exercises discourage congestion in the breasts by boosting the circulation of blood and lymph.

Massage – Anecdotal evidence suggests that breast play during love-making may help some lumpy breasts by decreasing congestion.

Hydrotherapy – Reduce any congestion by splashing your breasts each day with cold water for one minute, then hot water for half a minute, repeating this several times. Or spray them in the shower, alternately with a long spray of comfortably hot water and a quick spray of cold water.

Aromatherapy – Add a few drops of an oil reputed to help balance hormones (such as geranium, clary sage or rose), plus a 'calming' oil (such as lavender) to your bath water. Alternatively, add three or four drops of one of these oils to a tablespoon of sweet almond or other carrier oil for a gentle breast massage. Make this a part of love-play with your partner, or do it yourself. (Note the advice on page 288 concerning the use of essential oils.)

Herbal remedies – Try *Vitex agnus castus* for three months, or false unicorn root for the same time. (Note the advice on pages 277 and 286 concerning the use of herbal remedies.)

Tests and investigations

Your doctor will examine your breasts and may recommend a mammogram or ultrasound scan to check for breast cancer. Fluid can be drawn off a cyst via a needle aspiration in which a doctor passes a fine needle into the lump and uses a vacuum to draw out some cells; these can then be sent to a laboratory to be checked for cancer. Sometimes a surgical biopsy is necessary.

Medical treatment

There are several options, so talk to your doctor about the best way forward.

> **need to see a doctor?**
>
> See a doctor for new lumpiness; lumpiness that is different from usual for the time of month; any new lump that's large, hard, painful or unexpected; or any concern about a lump or other breast change. Also, ensure regular assessment of any continuing lump. Lumpiness on starting the Pill or HRT or changing to a different formulation is likely to settle in two to three months; if not, see a doctor.

- You could switch to a less oestrogenic type of Pill or HRT, use other contraception or stop HRT.

- A simple cyst can be drained through a needle – at the same time as a needle biopsy or if you simply wish to be rid of the lump. However, it's quite likely to fill again.

- Drug therapy can counteract lumpiness that continues to be painful or otherwise problematic. The choice is between danazol or gestrinone, or bromocriptine. All these can have side effects (see pages 302-303).

- A fibroadenoma is probably best surgically removed if you are over 30, or if your mother, sister or daughter has, or has had, breast cancer.

your action plan

Any lump or lumpiness

✔ **Vital**

- Breast awareness
- Healthy weight maintainance
- Right-size bra

✔ **Could be vital**

- Medical treatment

Benign breast changes

✔ **Vital**

- Discourage oestrogen dominance (page 89)
- Cut down on coffee, tea, cola, cocoa, and chocolate

(✔) **Optional**

- Massage • Hydrotherapy
- Aromatherapy • Herbal remedies

breast-skin changes

Almost any skin condition can affect the skin over the breasts, including eczema and other dermatitis, psoriasis, acne, soreness from rubbing or other injury, dryness, age spots, moles, melanomas, and fungal infections such as candida. Certain 'whole-body' rashes, such as measles, chickenpox and ringworm, can be to blame, as can the *Herpes zoster* infection called shingles. Sometimes breast cancer causes breast skin changes.

what to do yourself

If you know what's wrong, treat it with appropriate home remedies and over-the-counter drugs.

Watch out especially for:

• Patches of itchy allergic contact dermatitis due, for example, to nickel in metal bra fittings, exposed rubber in bra elastic, or traces of washing powder in your bra. Aim to identify and avoid the culprit.

• Sore skin beneath the breasts due to a tight bra, or a fungal and/or bacterial infection encouraged by warmth, high humidity, darkness, and overweight. Buy a better fitting bra; lose excess weight if necessary; wear a fresh bra each day; and twice a day wash and dry skin well, and apply undiluted tea-tree oil.

• Any hard, puckered, dimpled or abnormally coloured area; at worst, this could indicate an underlying cancer.

• Eczema of the nipple or areola; this is most often due to something reversible, such as contact dermatitis from a washing powder but could be caused by an abnormal discharge or even a cancer in a milk duct.

need to see a doctor?

Medical tests, investigations and treatments

Your doctor will diagnose the condition, recommend treatment, and do a breast-cancer check if necessary.

Yes, unless you know what's wrong and home treatment is successful.

symptom sorter

Gynae or gynae-related causes of breast skin changes

● ● ● **Most likely** – sex flush, indentation from tight bra, stretch marks, dermatitis, psoriasis, acne, injury, fungal infection (e.g. candida), 'whole-body' rash

● ● **Less likely** – dryness, sunburn, age spot, mole

● **Possible** – breast cancer

your action plan

✔ **Could be vital**
• Medical assessment
• Appropriate home and medical treatments

breast swelling

General swelling (as distinct from a lump or general lumpiness) is normal during sexual arousal, pregnancy and in a breastfeeding woman as her breasts fill with milk. Other common causes include weight gain and fluid retention. At other times swelling is often hormone-related, occurring before a period (perhaps as part of premenstrual syndrome), on the Pill, around the menopause or with HRT. Some women have enough swelling to warrant a bigger bra, or other symptoms – such as lumps, skin changes, and breast tenderness or pain. This may mean that their breasts are over-sensitive to normal levels of hormones or to changing hormone levels, or that they have an oestrogen-dominant hormone imbalance. Swelling can also result from a breast infection (infected mastitis) when accompanied by redness, pain, tenderness and a fever.

what to do yourself

If your breasts are unacceptably tense and uncomfortable, or you suspect something is wrong, the following should help:

Breast awareness – Keep a diary note of your periods, and daily estimates of the degree of swelling, and whether you are retaining fluid elsewhere – around your ankles and fingers, for example. This will suggest whether the swelling is hormone sensitive, or simply due to 'whole-body' weight gain – though this itself can increase oestrogen levels and thereby encourage hormone-sensitive breast swelling.

For hormone-sensitive swelling

Discourage oestrogen dominance – (see page 89).

Consider – using the advice on massage, herbal remedies, aromatherapy, and hydrotherapy under 'Breast lumps' on page 61.

need to see a doctor?

Yes, if your breasts are unacceptably tense or swollen and home remedies don't work; you're on the Pill or HRT; something else is wrong, such as a fever, redness of the skin, or a lump or only one breast is swollen.

Medical tests, investigations and treatments

Your doctor will examine your breasts, and arrange hormone tests, if necessary, to help work out the cause. You may need to discuss changing or coming off the Pill or HRT.

symptom sorter

Gynae or gynae-related causes of breast swelling

● ● ● **Most likely** – sexual arousal, normal premenstrual (and newborn) hormone changes, weight gain, pregnancy, presence of breast milk, the Pill, HRT

● ● **Less likely** – premenstrual syndrome, fluid retention, oestrogen dominance, oversensitivity to sex hormones or their changing levels

● **Possible** – breast infection, lymphoedema, large breast lump, breast implants

your action plan

For any swelling

✔ **Vital**

• Breast awareness

✔ **Could be vital**

• Medical assessment

Also, for hormone-sensitive swelling

✔ **Vital**

• Discourage oestrogen dominance (see page 89)

• Consider massage, herbal remedies, aromatherapy, and hydrotherapy

breast pain

Some women have cyclical pain with discomfort and, perhaps, lumpiness in both breasts before a period as part of benign breast changes but this usually disappears soon after bleeding begins. Sometimes pain occurs on starting the Pill, when pregnant, around the menopause, from oversensitivity to normal hormone changes, on starting HRT or from fluid retention due to an oestrogen-dominant hormone imbalance. It can also result from oestrogen deficiency.

Non-cyclical pain can affect one or both breasts and sometimes goes down the arm. It may be due to inflammation (mastitis – which, in a breastfeeding woman, could be associated with a blocked milk duct, infected mastitis or an abscess). A breastfeeding woman may also have tender breasts if she doesn't breastfeed (or express milk) often or efficiently enough. Two in five over-70s have a condition called duct ectasia in which the milk ducts under the areola are swollen and feel like lengths of thick string. This is usually not a problem but sometimes the ducts become inflamed, leading to tenderness or a dull, drawing pain and a discharge that may cause itching and burning around the nipple. Over the years, the dilated ducts tend to shorten, which may invert the nipples.

It's very unusual for pain to be the only sign of cancer and there need not be any pain at all. However, having breast pain doesn't preclude the possibility that you don't also have cancer.

what to do yourself

For any pain

Breast awareness – Keep a diary of periods and pain, as cyclical pain suggests it is hormone-sensitive.

Exercise – Do regular 'whole-body' aerobic exercise to boost your general health, and arm exercises (such as swinging them round and round and up and down) to discourage any congestion in the breasts.

Dietary changes – Try eating more foods rich in vitamin B (which sometimes eases breast pain), and selenium (as women with breast pain tend to be low on this mineral). Eat more foods rich in omega-3 fatty acids and less of those rich in omega-6s. A good balance of these fatty acids aids healthy hormone balance. Reduce your total intake of fat, especially saturated. Avoid foods made with white flour and sugar, to counteract fluid retention. (See pages 255-262 for dietary information.)

Go bra-less or get a better-fitting bra – One study suggests that this can reduce pain significantly, possibly because a tight bra blocks the flow of blood and lymph in certain parts of the breast.

For hormone-sensitive pain:

Lifestyle tips – Work out whether oestrogen dominance is likely; if so, use the tips on page 91. Also, use the tips on hydrotherapy, massage (if this helps), and aromatherapy, already mentioned for breast lumps (see pages 59-60).

Food supplements – Consider taking, for at least four months, fish oil, which contains two omega-3 fatty acids (docosahexaenoic and eicosapentanoic acids).

Herbal remedies – Consider taking red clover, *Vitex agnus castus*, false unicorn root, or black cohosh to relieve the pain. Note the advice on using these herbs on pages 277-286.)

For inflamed duct ectasia:

Dietary changes – Eat more foods rich in omega-3 fatty acids and less of those rich in omega-6s but reduce your total intake of fat, especially saturated fat, to reduce inflammation.

Heat – Use warmth, for example, from a hot compress or heated pad, to soothe pain.

Medical tests, investigations and treatments

Your doctor might do a breast-cancer check and arrange further tests, if necessary and discuss treatment. For hormone-sensitive pain this might mean changing or coming off the Pill or HRT or doing a three-month trial of danazol or bromocriptine. For infected mastitis, it means antibiotics. For inflamed duct ectasia with a discharge, it means having laboratory tests to see whether infection is present and, if so, which antibiotics are indicated. If inflamed duct ectasia continues to be a big problem a breast surgeon can remove the affected tissue and, if necessary, insert cosmetic implants.

need to see a doctor?

Yes, if you don't know what's wrong, or if the pain continues in spite of home treatments, or is sudden, severe, or combined with other symptoms, such as a fever. Also, get medical advice if you have inflamed duct ectasia, with painfully swollen milk ducts under the areola that feel like tender pieces of string.

symptom sorter

Gynae or gynae-related causes of breast pain or tenderness

● ● ● **Most likely** – oversensitivity to normal menstrual, pregnancy or menopausal hormone changes; HRT; benign breast changes; infrequent breastfeeding, a blocked milk duct, infected mastitis, or an abscess in a breastfeeding woman.

● ● **Less likely** – oestrogen dominance, oestrogen deficiency.

● **Possible** – injury, duct ectasia, breast cancer.

your action plan

Any pain

✔ **Vital**

• Breast awareness

✔ **Could be vital**

• Exercise
• Dietary changes
• Going bra-less or getting a better bra

Inflamed duct ectasia

✔ **Vital**

• Dietary changes

✔ **Could be vital**

• Medical treatment

(✔) **Optional**

• Heat

Hormone-sensitive pain

✔ **Vital**

• Breast awareness
• Dietary changes
• Healthy weight
• Exercise
• Stress management
• Bright daylight
• Avoiding non-essential antibiotics

✔ **Could be vital**

• Medical treatment

(✔) **Optional**

• Hydrotherapy
• Massage
• Food supplements
• Aromatherapy
• Herbal remedies

discontent with breast size

An increasing number of women today are opting for breast surgery to improve, as they perceive it, the appearance of their breasts.

what to do yourself

Don't waste money on creams claimed to enlarge small breasts, because there's no good evidence that they work. However, several things are worthwhile.

Positive thinking – Learn to be positive about yourself and your breasts. Every day, for example, tell yourself you are uniquely special, your breasts are beautiful as they are, and they certainly don't have to compete with others.

There is some evidence that **'visualisation'** – imagining, or picturing in your mind's eye, that you have larger breasts – helps them become larger. If this works, it's probably by increasing the blood flow to the breasts. It's harmless and you may think it's worth trying at least three months of twice daily 'treatment'.

Clothing tips – Experiment with clothes to see what flatters your figure. For example, if you have large breasts, wear garments with a waist (unless you are overweight, in which case you may prefer the look of long loose tops), steer clear of big patterns and enjoy low tops in the evening. If you have small breasts, try inserting shoulder pads into shirts and, perhaps, jumpers and jackets, avoid tight tops and choose a bra that's either padded or pushes the breasts together to give the impression of a natural cleavage.

Nutrition and exercise – If you have large breasts and are overweight, eat less, eat a healthy diet and exercise more, so as to lose some of the surplus from all over your body, including your breasts. If you have small breasts and are underweight, aim to gain some pounds by eating more and, again, eating a healthy diet. Whatever your weight, if you have small breasts, do upper body weight training to enlarge your pectoral muscles ('pecs'), as this will push your existing breast tissue out a little.

Good posture – Whatever your shape, stand up straight, especially if you have such heavy breasts that you get backache. One tip for good posture is to imagine you are a puppet controlled by a cord attached to the back of the top of your head.

69

Breastfeeding is possible after breast augmentation surgery and may even be possible after breast reduction surgery that involves repositioning the nipple and areola, since any severed breast ducts tend to join up again over the months.

need to see a doctor?

Yes, if you feel depressed and blame it on the shape of your breasts, because a discussion with your doctor, or a visit to a counsellor recommended, perhaps, by your doctor, may help you to put things into perspective and focus on what's really wrong. If you do want to explore further the idea of surgery to make your breasts bigger or smaller, be aware that although such operations are called 'cosmetic', they carry the same risks as any other surgery, including side effects from the general anaesthetic and post-operative infection. Also, breast implants can leak, burst or lead to hardening of surrounding breast tissue and quite a few women decide eventually to have them removed.

your action plan

✔ Vital
- Positive thinking
- Nutrition and exercise
- Good posture

(✔) Optional
- Visualisation
- Clothing tips
- Surgery

nipple itching and/or discharge

Some women's nipples normally tingle or itch before a period, during pregnancy or at the start of a breastfeed. Itching can also result from allergic or irritant contact dermatitis caused by something that touches your skin (such as traces of laundry products in the bra, nightdress or sheets, or certain creams, lotion, perfumes or drugs). A breastfeeding woman may get eczema from a product she's putting on her nipples or from traces of foods or medicaments in her baby's mouth. Another possibility is a fungal skin infection such as candida. Either condition could be weepy.

During pregnancy, a discharge could be colostrum (the earliest milk); during or after breastfeeding it could be milk. Many women who have breastfed sometimes find a little dried milk on their nipples, and are always able to express a few drops of milk.

A very few women who aren't pregnant or breastfeeding produce abnormal amounts of milk because their pituitary gland is producing too much prolactin. This can result from certain drugs (such as phenothiazines, taken, for example, for schizophrenia), a pituitary tumour, an underactive thyroid, an illness called sarcoidosis, and kidney failure. Stress can also sometimes increase the prolactin level. Other possible symptoms from too much prolactin include absent periods, fertility problems, weight gain, low sex drive, and a dry vagina; a tumour may also cause headaches and visual problems.

Other possibilities are a duct infection (producing a bloodstained, yellow or green discharge); a sore or cracked nipple while breastfeeding (producing a bloody discharge); a tumour called a papilloma in a milk duct; or a breast cancer. Itching and inflammation of one nipple are very occasionally early signs of a milk-duct cancer, and are known as Paget's disease of the nipple. Some older women have a condition called duct ectasia that can cause a discharge of thick, sticky, cheesy, pearly or multicoloured fluid; this may cause itching and burning around the nipple (see Breast pain, page 65).

what to do yourself

For contact dermatitis:

Aim to identify and avoid the trigger.

For fungal infection:

Tea tree oil or anti-fungal cream – Apply one or two drops of undiluted tea tree oil to each newly washed and dried nipple twice a day. If, after two or three days, you're no better, ask your pharmacist to recommend an anti-fungal cream. Treat any patches of infection elsewhere on your body, and organise treatment for those you live with if they have signs of infection anywhere.

Hot Laundry – Wear a fresh bra each day, laundered as hot as possible.

Anti-fungal diet – Avoid foods and drinks with added sugar and white flour. Eat differently coloured vegetables for a variety of natural antioxidants and anti-fungal agents. Consider consulting a nutritional therapist to improve your diet.

For inflamed duct ectasia:

See 'Breast pain', page 65.

For breast cancer:

See page 73.

> **need to see a doctor?**
>
> See your doctor for help with tests, diagnosis and treatment if you have itching, nipple 'eczema' that doesn't clear up, or an unusual discharge that doesn't respond to home treatment or if you notice unexplained blood or pus. If necessary, you can have skin tests for contact sensitivity, fungal testing of scraped off skin cells, bacterial testing of a discharge or a cancer check. A urine sugar test for diabetes is wise if a discharge is making you itch.

symptom sorter

Gynae or gynae-related causes of nipple itching and/or discharge

● ● ● **Most likely** – dermatitis; fungal infection (e.g. candida); sore or cracked nipple, or a milk-duct infection or abscess in a breastfeeding woman; high prolactin level (e.g. in late pregnancy, while breastfeeding, while taking phenothiazines); orgasm in a breastfeeding woman.

● ● **Less likely** – duct ectasia, milk-duct papilloma.

● **Possible** – breast cancer, Paget's disease of nipple.

your action plan

Contact dermatitis

✔ **Vital**

• Identify and avoid the trigger

✔ **Could be vital**

• Medical treatment

Fungal infection

✔ **Vital**

• Tea tree oil or anti-fungal cream

• Hot laundering

✔ **Could be vital**

• Anti-fungal diet

• Medical treatment

breast cancer

In the UK breast cancer affects one in nine women at some time in her life, in the USA, one in eight and the figure is on the increase (though this may be partly accountable to better detection). Thankfully, though, the number of women dying from breast cancer is going down. This cancer is the most common cancer in women, though it is not necessarily responsible for the most deaths. (In the UK, for example, more women die from lung cancer.) Most breast cancers start in a milk duct.

Factors that encourage it:

Age – one in five breast cancers occurs in women under 50, four in five women over 50. *Age is the only strong risk factor.*

Location – women in developed countries have a higher risk. Also, the latitude at which you live may affect how much light you get (see 'Lack of bright light', below).

Cancer in the other breast.

Previous benign breast lumps – those reported by the laboratory as having cells showing 'severe atypical epithelial hyperplasia' increase the risk most.

Ionising radiation – the risk to an older woman from a mammogram, for example, is very low, but a young woman's risk is slightly higher, which is partly why mammograms aren't routinely used for screening under-50s.

signs of breast cancer

- A lump in the breast, armpit, arm, or around the collarbone is the commonest sign.
- An area of skin hardening, thickening, puckering, dimpling or reddening.
- A retracted (also called inverted or indrawn) nipple.
- New veins that stand out, particularly on one breast only.
- A change in a breast's size or shape, or in the direction a nipple points.
- A rash or discolouration of the nipple or areola.
- Swelling of an arm (lymphoedema).
- Breast pain that's mainly in one part and doesn't go after a period.
- A bloodstained discharge from the nipple (this is rare).

A high lifetime number of ovulatory menstrual cycles – because the repeated hormone swings associated with these can disrupt breast cells. Several things increase this number, including starting periods particularly young. Not having children makes cancer 10-30 per cent more likely (the average woman's risk decreases by 8 per cent for each child). Having your first child in your 30s increases your risk of premenopausal cancer by 63 per cent and postmenopausal cancer by 35 per cent. Not breastfeeding each child relatively frequently, day and night raises the premenopausal cancer risk: the average woman's risk decreases by 4 per cent for each year of breastfeeding. This is because frequent breastfeeding delays the return of menstrual hormone swings after childbirth. Having your menopause over 55 makes cancer twice as likely as having it before 45.

A family history of breast, ovary or colon cancer – nearly 8 per cent of women whose mother, sister or daughter had early breast cancer develop the disease themselves; over 13 per cent of those with two close relatives and over 21 per cent with three. An heritable defect in the BRCA1 or 2, CHEK2, or other genes causes up to one in 20 of *all* breast cancers but as many as about a third of those in under-35s. Such defects also encourage ovary cancer. A woman with a BRCA defect has a 50% chance of developing breast cancer by 50 years old, and a 60-85% risk by 70.

The Pill – Older studies suggested there was a small risk that increased the longer you were on the Pill and tended to normalise once you were off the Pill for 10 years. However, a recent study has found that the Pill increases the risk only in under-30s whose mother or sister has had pre-menopausal breast cancer.

A lack of bright light – people living farthest from the equator have more than two-and-a-half times the risk of those nearer the equator. Scientists suspect this may be partly due to a lack of vitamin D, which helps to regulate cell division and so might limit cancer-cell multiplication. Certainly women with breast cancer are more likely to have a low level. Alternatively, the raised risk could be associated with a lack of melatonin, a very potent natural antioxidant hormone that may have anti-cancer properties and is produced by the pineal at night when it's dark. Women with oestrogen-sensitive breast cancer (see An oestrogen-dominant hormone imbalance, facing page) tend to have a low level of melatonin. Since bright light is needed to make a neurotransmitter called serotonin from which the pineal produces melatonin, it's possible, though unproven, that getting too little bright light – for example, by living far from the equator – could encourage breast cancer. To make enough melatonin you need enough bright light *and* enough darkness in each 24-hour day. Interestingly, breast cancer is most often diagnosed in winter. The raised risk of breast cancer in long-haul air-crew and frequent flyers may be due to jet lag lowering melatonin production by disturbing the sleep-wake cycle. However, exposure to ionising radiation at high altitudes could also be to blame. Finally, there's some evidence that UV may encourage cancer cells to 'commit suicide' (a normal and valuable cellular process called apoptosis).

Being overweight and post-menopausal – obesity is the most important known reason in this age group for high levels of oestrogen and testosterone and a recent study found that older women who have high levels of these hormones have twice the risk of breast cancer as those with low levels. If you are pre-menopausal, however, being overweight actually reduces your risk of breast cancer.

High socio-economic group – women in higher-earning and professional households have a higher risk.

An unhealthy diet – research suggests that this encourages four in every five cancers; even just one helping a day of fresh vegetables seems to reduce the risk by over 20 per cent, for example.

More than one unit of alcohol a day on a regular basis. An analysis of many studies clearly links alcohol with a raised risk of breast cancer. Any intake encourages cancer, and the more alcohol you drink, the higher the risk, though this risk is small. More worrying is that young women who drink too much dramatically increase their risk. Just one unit of alcohol a day for young women raises the risk by 9 per cent; up to 14 units a week, by 20 per cent and regular binge drinking (more than four units in a session) by up to 40 per cent.

An oestrogen-dominant hormone imbalance – Four in five breast cancers are made of cells containing oestrogen receptors, which means they are sensitive to oestrogen, and oestrogen stimulates them to multiply. Many of the other risk factors mentioned act by encouraging oestrogen-dominant hormone imbalance. About 60 per cent of breast cancers in premenopausal women are 'oestrogen-receptor positive' or oestrogen-sensitive (and about 75 per cent in postmenopausal women). Most cancers associated with BRCA gene defects are oestrogen-receptor negative.

HRT – evidence suggests that this increases the risk and that the risk becomes higher the longer you are on it. Women who develop breast cancer on HRT usually have the oestrogen-sensitive type. However, the effect is small; fatal breast cancer is less likely and the risk normalises once you have been off it for five years.

Lack of exercise – regular exercise boosts immunity.

Smoking – although some evidence has suggested that both smoking and passive smoking increase the risk, the largest and most recent study has found this not to be so.

Repeated use of dark brown or black hair dye

At least six studies over the years suggest that the regular long-term use of hair dye encourages breast cancer. (It has also been associated with cancers of the ovary, bladder, lymph system, bone marrow and white blood cells – leukaemia). However, several other studies have found no link with breast cancer – so, although the design of these particular studies has been criticised, the jury is still out. Until scientists have more definite information many people think it is wise to err on the side of caution by avoiding colouring their hair regularly and frequently (for example, every four to six weeks) for years with permanent or semi-permanent brown or black hair dyes..

Scientists don't know which, if any, dye chemicals encourage cancer from normal use but they are suspicious of several, including para-phenylenediamine and toluenediamine and tetrahydro-6-nitroquinoxaline. All dyes contain similar chemicals, but darker colours have greater concentrations, so more is absorbed. 'Permanent' ('level 3') colours have higher concentrations than 'tone on tone' or 'demi-permanents' ('level 2', lasting up to 24 washes), which in turn have higher ones than 'semi-permanents' ('level 1', lasting up to 6-8 washes). Note that permanent 'vegetable' or 'herbal' dyes may contain one of the chemicals under suspicion.

In contrast, bleach (hydrogen peroxide) is not under suspicion; nor are 'colour restorers' that gradually darken hair or temporary-colour rinses (wash-in, wash-out), sprays or mousses.

If you decide to go on using hair dye, always follow the instructions – for example wear gloves, don't leave the dye on for too long and rinse well.

Until we know more, you may also want to take the following precautions:

• If you've been using black or dark-brown dye, gradually go lighter, and favour level 1 or 2 products if practicable.

• If you aren't yet going grey, consider having 'highlights' or 'lowlights' rather than all-over colour, as the foil-wrapping process involved means dye does not touch the scalp.

• If you are dark-haired but going grey, use a level 2 or 3 product that is lighter than your original colour, and have bleached highlights or lowlights put in to soften the junction with the new grey growth; you may then get away with colouring roots less often.

what to do yourself

To help prevent breast cancer

Be breast aware (see page 60).

Have any necessary screening (pages 46-56).

Avoid or minimise risk factors, see above, wherever possible.

Discourage oestrogen dominance (see page 89) if you have cyclical symptoms (such as lumpiness), since these could result from oestrogen dominance that would encourage oestrogen-sensitive breast cancer. Dietary changes (see page 255), alcohol awareness, healthy weight maintenance, regular exercise, avoidance of xeno-oestrogens (see page 39) and getting enough bright light and darkness are all useful.

Other dietary changes

It seems wise to eat more foods rich in plant oestrogens. In one recent study of Chinese women in Singapore, for example, those who ate plenty of food made from soy beans were 60 per cent less likely than those who ate very little of this food to develop changes in their mammograms linked with a high risk of breast cancer. In another study 28 US nuns aged 65 or over tested the effects of ground linseeds, which contain higher quantities of those plant oestrogens called lignans than any other food. Some ate 5 or 10 grams a day for seven weeks, the others none. Blood tests showed that the levels of certain sex hormones that can be associated with breast cancer were lower in those who had eaten the linseeds. Whether this was due to plant oestrogens or other constituents of linseeds is unclear, as is whether linseeds help prevent breast cancer. But it does no harm to eat a daily tablespoon – perhaps added to cereal, casseroles, sauces or fruit 'smoothies'. Grind the seeds first, or eat ready-cracked ones (check on the packet), or you won't digest them.

Have plenty of calcium. Most women's main source is dairy food. It has been suggested that dairy food may encourage breast cancer, however, recent research has found no significant association between dairy-food intake and breast cancer.

Also, include tomatoes in your diet – sometimes cooked in olive oil or other fat, as this raises their content of lycopene, a potent carotenoid antioxidant, and eat plenty of foods rich in folic acid and other B vitamins.

Take general anti-cancer measures (See 'Gynae cancers' page 84).

Alcohol – Clearly it's wise to stick to recommended limits. But if other factors are also increasing your breast-cancer risk – and especially if your doctor considers your risk very high – you may opt to drink even less alcohol or perhaps none at all.

Watch your weight – Being overweight makes breast cancer harder to detect. This cancer is also more common in overweight postmenopausal women. If you can't lose weight and keep it off, be sure to eat a healthy diet; your body needs more nutrients to keep the increased bulk healthy. And never put off having a mammogram because you are embarrassed about your size.

Get enough light and dark – This may be particularly important if you live in a northern latitude, work at night, have a dark skin, or wear clothes that cover almost all your skin.

To help treat breast cancer (in addition to having medical treatment)

Use all of the above tips, as they may help you to feel better, prevent the development of new cancers and slow the growth of certain cancers.

Discouraging oestrogen dominance is particularly important if your breast cancer is oestrogen-sensitive. If you don't know, ask your doctor whether lab tests have shown it to be 'oestrogen-receptor positive' ('E-R positive' – E for 'estrogen'). If so, oestrogen dominance could encourage it to grow.

Friendship, stress management, laughter and enjoyment – One US study found that the more close friends a woman with breast cancer had, the less likely the cancer was to kill her. In another study, involving nearly 400 women free from breast cancer for an average of nine years, 42 per cent believed stress had been a main cause (compared with 27 per cent who blamed genes, 26 per cent environmental factors, 24 per cent hormones and 16 per cent diet) and 60 per cent felt that a positive attitude had kept their cancer away. However, other evidence suggests that if stress is a contributory factor in breast cancer, it is not a significant one. Of course, a positive attitude does help a woman to feel more in control, which could, in turn, help her to maintain proven helpful behaviours, such as exercising more and eating a healthy diet.

Exercise – One study found that when women who were on chemotherapy, radiotherapy or hormone treatment for early breast cancer, walked for an hour three to five times a week, they felt better.

To help treat lymphoedema

Some women with breast cancer develop lymphoedema – swelling of the arm and hand (and, perhaps, breast) on the side of the cancer, though changes in surgical technique mean that this is less likely nowadays. It results from mastectomy or radiotherapy damaging the lymph vessels, or from cancer cells invading the armpit's lymph nodes ('glands'). The swelling results from restriction of the flow of lymph (a fluid that travels from around the cells, where it's called 'tissue fluid', into vessels that carry lymph up the arm to the chest and then into the bloodstream). When a lymph vessel is blocked, lymph and tissue fluid accumulate in the arm and hand, making them painful, heavy, hard and itchy, restricting movement, and encouraging skin damage.

A regular special lymph-drainage massage by a therapist trained in this technique can help, or you could learn to do a simple version yourself. Care for your skin well, and wear an elastic sleeve by day, and, perhaps, a bandage by night. Don't let anyone take your blood pressure or a blood sample or give you an injection, in that arm, as this could encourage infection.

Tests and investigations

Your doctor will examine you and, if necessary, arrange a mammogram and/or ultrasound or MRI (magnetic resonance imaging) scan and a biopsy of any lump.

Medical treatment

The choice depends on the nature of your cancer, and your health and medical and family history. The possibilities include:

Surgery

The trend today is to preserve as much of the breast as possible, and to follow surgery with radiotherapy.

Lumpectomy (lump removal) is recommended for at least 60-70 per cent of women, in whom

need to see a doctor?

Women with a very high risk (see pages 73-76) benefit from having more frequent screening mammograms. Report any unexplained breast symptoms (see page 73) early, because if you have a cancer, the smaller it is when it's first treated, the better. For example, in the UK, 9 in 10 women with a cancer less than 2cm (⅘ inch) across when first treated are alive five years later, as compared with only 6 in 10 whose cancer was bigger than 5cm (2in). The average five-year survival from breast cancer is 75 per cent in the UK and about 85 per cent in Australia and the USA.

the cancer can be removed with around 1cm (⅘ inch) of healthy breast tissue around it, enabling a good cosmetic result. The surgeon will either take a biopsy from one of the underarm lymph nodes ('glands') so the laboratory can examine it for cancer cells or remove these nodes.

Mastectomy (breast removal) is now recommended for 30-40 per cent of women at most. The options are a 'simple' mastectomy; a 'modified radical' mastectomy (removal of the breast plus the underarm nodes – 'glands' – on that side) and a 'radical' mastectomy (removal of the breast, surrounding chest muscles and underarm lymph nodes). Reconstruction of the breast can be done immediately, using skin and muscle from your back. Recovery takes up to six weeks.

Studies suggest that if you are premenopausal and have a hormone-sensitive cancer, surgery may be most successful on days 1-2 or 13-32 of your menstrual cycle (the first day of a period being day 1).

Post-operative radiotherapy

Small doses of radiation to the site where the cancer was are usually given in five sessions a week for five weeks with a further week's treatment later. The aim is to destroy any cancer cells that may remain. It reduces local cancer recurrence by around 20-30 per cent. Surprisingly, though, it has little effect on long term survival.

Drugs

These may also be given after surgery to destroy any cancer cells that may remain and to lessen the risk of a return or spread. The two main types of drug treatment are chemotherapy and hormone therapy (sometimes these are used together). 'Biological therapy' is a newer treatment (see below).

Chemotherapy. This treatment with drugs that destroy cancer cells is generally recommended after surgery for premenopausal women; sometimes, though, it is used to shrink a cancer before surgery.

Hormone therapy. These therapies target oestrogen-sensitive cancers.

• Tamoxifen is a hormone-like drug that attaches itself to oestrogen receptors on breast cancer cells, partially blocking them and so helping to prevent a woman's oestrogen from stimulating cancer growth. Many over-55s with breast cancer now have this drug for up to five years, not only those with a positive oestrogen-receptor test (because such tests aren't foolproof). Tamoxifen reduces mortality from breast cancer by up to 30 per cent; reduces recurrence of the cancer by around 50 per cent and reduces the risk of cancer in the other breast by around 40 per cent.

• Aromatase inhibitors (anastrozole, letrozole and formestane) can help to treat oestrogen-sensitive cancer, help to prevent the recurrence of oestrogen-sensitive cancer and help to prevent cancer in the other breast. This is because they reduce oestrogen production by blocking the action of aromatase – the enzyme in fat cells and ovaries that changes androgens such as testosterone to oestrogen and is the main source of oestrogen after the menopause. They also cause hot flushes and nausea in some women.

• Artificial menopause – Drugs that cause an artificial menopause are useful for some premenopausal women with oestrogen-sensitive cancer. Drugs called gonadotrophin-releasing-hormone analogues (such as goserelin) lower the pituitary gland's production of the body's own gonadotrophins, and hence lower the ovaries'

prevention of breast cancer in high-risk women

Prevention of breast cancer in high-risk women

Some opt to take tamoxifen as a preventive measure, Interestingly, trials suggest tamoxifen may also help to prevent primary breast cancer in women with a high risk due to having a mother, sister or daughter with pre-menopausal breast cancer.

A few high-risk women even opt to have their breasts removed.

new treatments

The search continues for better treatments. Two promising ones include:

Radiation inside the breast during lumpectomy: this involves 25 minutes of radiation from a device placed where the lump was. The idea is that this will kill off any remaining cancer cells and obviate the need for radiotherapy.

A breast-cancer vaccine (HER-2 DNA AutoVac): this 'therapeutic' vaccine (meaning one aiming to treat breast cancer, not prevent it) is being tested for advanced breast cancer. The aim is to stimulate the production of antibodies and 'killer cells' that target breast cancer.

oestrogen production to menopausal levels; they do this by 'downregulating' the pituitary – first stimulating then reducing gonadotrophin production. When you stop taking these drugs, your ovaries should work normally again. Surgical removal, or radiotherapy, of the ovaries also reduces oestrogen but their effects are permanent. They help around 30 per cent of premenopausal women.

Biological therapy. This is done with a 'drug' consisting of 'monoclonal' antibodies made in the laboratory. Its name is rastuzumab (trade name Herceptin) and it can help kill cancer cells which over-express (have too many) receptors for human epidermal growth factor (HER2); such over-expression happens in up to 30 per cent of cancers. This therapy also interferes with the development of the new blood vessels needed by the cancer to grow.

your action plan

✔ Vital
- Medical treatment
- Reduce controllable risk factors (see pages 73-77)

✔ Could be vital
- Discourage oestrogen dominance (see above and page 89)
- Dietary changes (see page 77)

- General anti-cancer measures (see page 84)
- Limit alcohol
- Light and dark exposure (see page 290)
- Healthy-weight maintenance
- Positive thinking, friends, stress management (see page 266), enjoyment

general gynae conditions

This section provides general information on gynae cancers – meaning cancers of the breast, ovary, womb, cervix and vulva (though each of these cancers is also considered individually elsewhere) and there are also entries on oestrogen dominance (a condition mentioned many times throughout the book), and oestrogen deficiency.

'gynae' cancers

Cancer results from damage to one or more of a cell's genes, making it prone to multiply in an uncontrolled way and form a malignant growth or 'cancer'. Depending on the gene damaged, a cell may be prevented from dying at its allotted time (as normal cells do). Genetic damage might also make cancer cells invisible to the immune system; encourage the development of the new blood vessels needed to nourish any cancer larger than a peppercorn or encourage cancer cells to spread via the bloodstream.

A cancer's growth rate depends on the genes affected, the cancer's type and stage and, for some, on certain environmental, lifestyle, hormonal and immunological factors. Dietary influences are often very important and long-term inflammation and/or infection – associated with disturbed immunity – are said to account for around one in three cancers.

Without treatment, a cancer can grow and destroy adjacent tissues. Cancer cells can also break away, travel in the blood or lymph and, unless destroyed by immune cells or by medical treatment, cause growths elsewhere ('secondaries' or metastases) that cause further damage. Eventually it can be fatal (unless it's so slow growing that a person dies of something else). The good news is that improvements in treatment mean that increasing numbers of people are living as cancer survivors.

what to do yourself

There's some evidence that the following natural treatments may help to prevent certain cancers or even to slow their growth, make them shrink, or prevent relapses, though they are not a cure as such. Even for people with advanced cancer, natural treatments occasionally prolong life by a short but precious time and improve its quality. They may help to prevent recurrence of cancer in survivors or the growth of new cancers. These treatments won't hurt and may make you feel better in yourself, so it's well worth using them alongside medical treatment.

General anti-cancer measures

Ensure that you have any screening recommended for your age or circumstances (see pages 46-56).

Reduce any controllable risk factors (see entry for each cancer).

Make dietary changes – Many cancers (including up to 80 per cent of breast cancers) may be preventable by dietary changes. Studies done in humans or in the test tube suggest that certain foods and nutrients are well worth including in your diet:

- Foods rich in **antioxidants** (page 259) help to prevent the free radicals that may encourage new cancer cells to develop and may help to destroy cancer cells. There's considerable interest in an antioxidant called inositol (which is related to vitamin B), as it's thought to help prevent cancer growth and shrink some cancers.

- Having at least five helpings of **vegetables and fruit** a day helps to prevent some cancers.

- **Ginger** and **turmeric** supply helpful antioxidants: curcumin in turmeric is thought to have tumour-suppressing properties.

- Beans contain **protease inhibitors** which may make it harder for cancer cells to invade nearby tissue.

- Beans and certain other foods, such as root vegetables and wholegrains (see page 260), contain **plant oestrogens**. Japanese women whose traditional diet is rich in plant oestrogens have a low risk of breast cancer. It's possible, though not proven, that dietary plant oestrogens help prevent oestrogen-sensitive cancer both in premenopausal women and in overweight post-menopausal women – as they have relatively high oestrogen levels for their stage of life. It's also possible that in women with oestrogen-sensitive cancer, dietary plant oestrogens help to slow its growth, and prevent its spread. However, until more is known about this, it's wise for women who have a personal or family history of such a cancer not to 'overdose' on plant oestrogens. This means not drinking litres of soybean milk each day, or taking a concentrated-soy supplement, though a diet naturally rich in plant hormones is considered safe.

• **Tomatoes** have more of a potent red carotene-like pigment called lycopene than any other vegetable, especially when cooked in olive oil or other fat. Lycopene has a very powerful anti-oxidant action, which means it can help dampen a chemical process called oxidation that may be associated with cancer.

• Powerful anti-cancer substances, such as glucosinolates, in **cruciferous vegetables** (cabbage, broccoli, brussels sprouts, kale, spring greens), may help to kill genetically damaged cells, so it's worth eating these vegetables several times a week

• S-allomercaptocysteine, found in cooked or raw **garlic**, is a natural cancer inhibitor; **onions** contain similar substances.

• **Citrus peel oil** contains powerful anti-cancer substances such as limonene (which is partly responsible for the bitter taste) and citrus flesh is a good source of vitamin C and flavonoids. So consider drinking each day a whole citrus fruit liquidised with its peel, and diluted if necessary.

• **Grapeskins** contain resveratrol, which can inhibit all stages of cancer growth, and ellagic acid, which blocks an enzyme cancer cells need to multiply.

• **Strawberries, cranberries, raspberries, blackberries, blueberries and cherries** contain cancer-fighting substances such as ellagic acid (see grapeskins, above)

• Foods rich in **salicylates** (fruits – especially their peel, vegetables, seeds, nuts) contain natural substances partially resembling aspirin, that may inhibit the production of prostaglandins that stimulate cancer growth and suppress immunity; they may also encourage certain cancer cells to 'commit suicide'.

• Foods rich in **fibre** may help to prevent oestrogen-sensitive cancer by lowering a raised oestrogen level. Also, a high-fibre diet is rich in a B vitamin called inositol that helps slow cancer growth.

• Polyphenols (such as tannic acid, epigallocatechin gallate, and theophylline) in **green tea** encourage the death of cells with damaged DNA.

• Eat more foods rich in **omega-3 fatty acids** and less of those rich in omega-6s (see page 256). A good balance of omega-3s and omega-6s enables normal serotonin production (which helps you to feel better) and a normal prostaglandin-balance (which boosts immunity, and helps to prevent inflammation). Research shows that one omega-3 fatty acid (eicosapentanoic acid) in oily fish aids weight gain in people who are losing weight because of cancer.

• Check that you have plenty of **zinc**-rich foods (see page 259), as zinc may help to prevent cancer and encourage better immunity.

• Note that foods made with white flour and sugar (which are refined carbohydrates), provide 'empty calories', meaning they lack the nutrients in whole foods and spoil your appetite for foods that are more nutrient-rich.

Supplements – There is some evidence that supplements of vitamins A and E or selenium may help to prevent certain cancers but the evidence isn't good enough to warrant a medical recommendation. If you do take supplements, avoid high doses. Also, avoid beta-carotene if you are a smoker, as studies suggest it encourages lung cancer and suppresses the production of certain of the body's natural antioxidants.

Keep to a healthy weight – Researchers believe that this could prevent one in six gynae cancers by discouraging oestrogen dominance. It may also help to slow the growth of an existing cancer, by reducing the level of a natural substance in the body called insulin-like growth factor.

Be alcohol-aware – Keep within recommended alcohol limits. (However, it's possible that antioxidants called catechins in wine help to prevent some cancers.)

Ensure enough exposure to light and darkness – Bathe in bright outdoor daylight for half an hour a day (without burning). This helps your hypothalamus to balance your hormone levels. It also boosts immunity by lifting your spirits (partly because it boosts serotonin), and it triggers vitamin D production, which is one reason why it's thought to help prevent cancer of the breast, ovaries, womb or cervix. (This also raises the possibility that it might aid treatment.) In winter in very northerly or southerly latitudes, consider using a light visor or box each day.

Getting enough bright light also enables your body to make serotonin and store it. If you get enough sleep in the dark, your body uses stored serotonin to make melatonin, a potent antioxidant that may help to prevent cancer. Boost melatonin production further by encouraging a good sleep-wake cycle – sleep in the dark at night, stay awake in the light by day, and get plenty of bright light, especially in the morning.

Identify any food sensitivity – It has been suggested, though it's completely unproven, that cancer may stop growing or even shrink when no longer exposed to certain foods to which an individual is sensitive. (One suggested culprit is a family of substances called lectins, present in many foods, including wheat, potatoes, tomatoes and peanuts.)

Exercise – Daily aerobic exercise helps to prevent cancer.

Several small studies suggest that regular exercise makes people with cancer feel better and less tired; some also note a lower risk of dying from cancer. But moderation is important, and it's wise to get your doctor's blessing.

Use effective stress management (see page 266) – Chronic long-term stress encourages cancer recurrence, probably because it reduces the activity of natural killer cells.

Positive thinking, friendship, meditation, laughter and enjoyment – Several studies suggest that people with cancer who think positively may live longer and although other studies have not found this to be so, there is no harm in trying. Some people find it helps them to think positively if they spend a few minutes each day on a 'visualisation' in which they imagine their immune cells are successfully destroying their cancer. Meditation may increase the melatonin level, which might help to prevent some cancers. Good social support can reduce stress, which may improve immunity and make cancer less likely to recur.

Self-help groups and cancer charities – These can empower you to help manage cancer.

Massage and aromatherapy – Gentle massage encourages relief from physical and mental tension, enables emotional release and helps you to feel cared for. One study found the physical and emotional benefits to be slightly enhanced when aromatherapy oils are used. Check with your doctor before having a massage.

Consider herbal remedies – Although good studies into the effects of herbal remedies in people with cancer are lacking, herbs that may boost immunity include echinacea, astragalus and burdock (astragalus may help check cancer spread). Test-tube experiments show that liquorice, silymarin (milk thistle), and burdock have anti-cancer properties; one important component of burdock, benzaldehyde, is also present in plum, apricot, peach and bitter almond kernels.

Essiac (named for the surname of its creator, Rene Caisse, spelt backwards; see Flor-Essence in the Helplist, page 315) is a mixture of extracts of burdock root, Indian rhubarb, sheep sorrel and the inner bark of slippery elm, watercress, blessed thistle, red clover and kelp. In 1993 the Canadian Breast Cancer Research Initiative said there was enough evidence of its beneficial effects to warrant further evaluation. Proponents claim Essiac is compatible with conventional cancer therapies.

Note the cautions in the section starting on page 274.

To help prevent hair loss from anti-cancer chemotherapy – If your cancer is to be treated with a drug that could make your hair fall out (visit www.cancernet.co.uk/hairloss.htm for a list of these) ask your cancer specialist whether the hospital offers 'head cooling'. The aim of this is to reduce or prevent hair loss and the success rate with certain drugs is up to 89 per cent. It's done by cooling the scalp during the administration of a drug, to constrict the blood vessels that supply the hair follicles and to reduce the metabolic rate of follicle cells; this reduces the amount of drug the follicle cells receive.

One concern is whether this might prevent enough of the drug from reaching any cancer cells that have strayed to the scalp, so it is not recommended if your cancer has spread from its primary site.

There are two methods of head cooling. One is to wear a 'cool cap'. This may be filled with gel that's been cooled in a freezer; be attached to a refrigeration unit that circulates coolant into it or be a home-made version improvised with bags of crushed ice. The other method is to sit under a hairdresser-style hood that blows cold air. The length of cooling time depends on the drug, and should also be one hour longer if your ethnic origin is Afro-Caribbean. A gel- or ice-filled cold cap must be changed every 20-40 minutes as it warms up. (See the Helplist on page 314 for suppliers of cooling systems.)

Researchers are currently developing a hair gel containing a substance which it is hoped will reduce hair loss by temporarily preventing cell division in hair follicles.

Other measures – There is much interest in certain other substances or therapies – including remedies made from shark cartilage, Gerson therapy (a programme of intensive nutrition, 'detoxification' and supplementation) and acupuncture – as possible anti-cancer agents. However, they are expensive and/or time consuming, and there is only anecdotal or early evidence, not high quality proof (with prospective randomised, controlled, double-blind clinical trials), that they are likely to help.

Tests and investigations

The choice, if any of these are necessary, depends on your symptoms (see the relevant sections on individual cancers).

need to see a doctor?

Always report any unexplained or worsening symptoms early, because the smaller a cancer is when it's first treated, the better.

Medical treatment

With treatment, many women survive cancer and die in old age of something unrelated. The 'five-year survival figure' – the number of women alive five years after their cancer diagnosis – is one often quoted indication of likely success, though the figure for any particular cancer varies in different countries and different centres and according to a woman's age and her cancer's stage and grade.

The choice of treatment depends on the nature and stage of the cancer, your age and health and the available health-care resources and includes various drugs, radiotherapy, and surgery.

your action plan

✔ **Vital**
• General anti-cancer measures (see above)
• Medical treatment

oestrogen dominance

This oestrogen/progesterone hormone imbalance (also called hyperoestrogenism) is relatively common in developed countries because of our typical unhealthy Western lifestyle, which encourages hormone-unfriendly hazards such as a poor diet, overweight and inactivity.

Possible gynae problems associated with oestrogen dominance include lumpy, painful, tender, swollen breasts; heavy and/or irregular periods; an abnormally thickened womb lining (endometrial hyperplasia); a vaginal discharge; polycystic ovary syndrome; infertility; repeated miscarriage; fibroids; endometriosis; cervical erosion; post-menopausal bleeding; and womb, ovary and breast cancer. It may also show up with weight gain, bloating, nausea and irritability.

Oestrogen dominance has three possible causes:

1   **You have too much oestrogen compared with progesterone.**

This may be because:

•   Egg follicles develop each month, but you don't ovulate – so there's no corpus luteum (see page 21) to raise the progesterone level in the second half of the cycle; this is a type of 'luteal defect'. Absent or irregular ovulation can happen for some months or years when periods first start in adolescence, for a few months after childbirth (longer if breastfeeding frequently) and for some months or years before the menopause. It can also result from severe stress, very rapid weight loss, being very underweight, bingeing, coming off the Pill, miscarriage and termination.

•   Your corpus luteum isn't producing enough progesterone.

•   Your ovaries, adrenal glands, and/or fat cells produce too much oestrogen, perhaps because you are overweight, eat a poor diet, don't exercise enough, make too much testosterone or have an ovary or adrenal tumour or an oestrogen-producing ovary cyst.

•   You are on the Pill or HRT.

2   **Your cells are unusually 'sensitive' to oestrogen (see page 16) or unusually insensitive to progesterone.**

3   **A relatively large proportion of the oestrogen in your blood is 'free'.**

Normally, if there's too much oestrogen in the blood, it's 'mopped up' by sex-hormone binding globulin (SHBG). However, SHBG production (by the liver) is reduced in women who are very overweight, have a high testosterone or low thyroid hormone level or take progestogens (as in the Pill or HRT), which frees up more oestrogen.

Another way in which the ovaries, womb and breasts can be affected by 'too much' oestrogen is if there's repeated oestrogenic stimulation from menstrual cycles occurring repeatedly for most of a woman's reproductive life. This may be particularly likely to cause problems if there is also oestrogen dominance in each cycle. It encourages several gynae disorders, including breast lumps, ovary cysts, and breast and ovary cancers.

what to do yourself

Dietary changes – Eat more fibre and less fat (especially saturated), as this reduces the numbers of those gut bacteria that produce beta-glucuronidase, an enzyme which enables oestrogen to be reabsorbed from the bowel to the blood.

Eat more foods rich in B vitamins, as these also encourage the liver to break down surplus oestrogen. Include yoghurt, as lactobacilli can help to lower the oestrogen level.

Eat beans, peas, lentils, onions and garlic; all of which are high in methionine, a sulphur-containing amino acid that helps the liver to break down excess oestradiol (the most potent form of a woman's oestrogen) into oestriol (a weaker sort).

Include other foods rich in plant oestrogens (see page 260) – again, pulses are good. These can reduce the oestrogenic activity of your own stronger oestrogens by occupying oestrogen receptors. They can also reduce the rate at which testosterone is converted into oestrogen in fat, and make oestrogen less available to cells. However, until we have more evidence about their safety, it's wise if you have a personal or family history of such a cancer not to 'overdose' on them (for example, by drinking litres of soy milk each day, or taking a concentrated-soy supplement).

Include in your diet some bitter foods or drinks (such as watercress, chicory, young dandelion leaves, rosemary, and tonic water) as these stimulate the liver and help it break down surplus oestrogen.

Eat cruciferous vegetables (such as cabbage, brussels sprouts, and cauliflower). These contain substances that stimulate the liver to break down surplus oestrogen into a water-soluble form the kidneys can excrete; inhibit the action of oestrogen and may inhibit the growth of breast-cancer cells.

Include fish, shellfish and, if you're a vegetarian, seaweed, in your diet, as these are rich sources of iodine. Most of us get enough iodine from vegetables and cereals, but a few don't – especially if they eat only produce grown locally in an area where the earth is low in iodine. An iodine deficiency can raise the oestrogen level by stimulating the sex hormone glands. However, avoid eating iodine-containing foods in the same meal as cruciferous vegetables, as these can reduce the uptake of iodine from your gut.

Drink only moderate amounts of alcohol; as little as three to six glasses of wine a week, for example, is enough to raise the oestrogen level.

Exercise – Take regular exercise as this reduces the rate of oestrogen production, but avoid too much exercise, as this could discourage ovulation.

Healthy weight maintenance – This is important, as oestrogen is produced in body fat by the action of an enzyme (aromatase) on testosterone. Too much fat around your middle is particularly likely to raise your oestrogen level. However, it is also important to remember that being too slim prevents ovulation.

No smoking – Smoking can damage arteries, which may discourage ovulation.

Stress management – If effective, this encourages ovulation – which helps to prevent oestrogen dominance in the second half of the cycle. It also aids healthy weight maintenance.

Exposure to light – Half an hour of bright outdoor daylight each day helps the hypothalamus to balance hormone levels.

Avoid exposure to xeno-oestrogens (see page 39).

Herbal remedies – Herbs that contain plant oestrogens and other hormone balancing herbs, may be helpful. See the entries on individual gynae conditions for suggestions as well as the advice about herbal remedies in Part Three.

Tests and investigations

These depend on your symptoms, since oestrogen dominance can be associated with so many gynae problems (see page 295).

Medical treatment

This is chosen according to the problem. For heavy periods associated with oestrogen

need to see a doctor?

Yes, if home treatments don't help your symptoms; if your symptoms are severe, or worsening; or you suspect you have a gynae cancer or other disorder.

dominance, your doctor may recommend a progestogen-releasing intra-uterine system (see page 43) or the combined contraceptive Pill; and for oestrogen-sensitive breast cancer, an 'anti-oestrogen' drug called tamoxifen (see page 308).

your action plan

✔ **Vital**

- Dietary changes
- Exercise
- Healthy weight maintenance
- No smoking
- Stress management
- Exposure to light

✔ **Could be vital**

- Avoiding exposure to xeno-oestrogens

(✔) **Optional**

- Herbal remedies

oestrogen deficiency

Possible gynae problems arising from an oestrogen-deficient hormone imbalance include irregular periods, painful and tender breasts, non-cyclical weight gain, infertility, a low sex drive, depression, fatigue, a dry vagina, acne, greasy hair and skin and unusual hairiness (for example, on the face and neck, and around the areolae).

It has three possible causes:

1   **You have too little oestrogen.**

This may be because:

- Your egg follicles aren't developing properly and you aren't ovulating, possibly as a result of severe stress, rapid weight loss or being very underweight.

- Your oestrogen production has fallen as a natural result of the menopause and subsequent ageing.

2   **Your cells are relatively insensitive to oestrogen.**

3   **A relatively large proportion of the oestrogen in your blood is bound rather than free.** This can happen if an unusually high level of sex-hormone binding globulin in the blood has 'mopped up' much of the free oestrogen, as can happen with a high thyroid hormone level.

what to do yourself

Dietary changes – A healthy diet helps to maintain a normal oestrogen level. Include plenty of foods rich in beta-carotene: the body makes this into vitamin A, which decreases the activity of an enzyme (beta-dehydrogenase) needed by the ovaries for oestrogen production. Also, have plenty of plant-oestrogen-rich food.

Avoid too much fibre, as this can increase the amount of oestrogen excreted in the bowel motions (see page 91).

Healthy weight maintenance – Avoid becoming too thin, as this can reduce ovary-stimulating hormone production by the pituitary gland.

No smoking – Smoking encourages the production of less active forms of oestrogen and encourages an early menopause.

Exercise – Try exercising less, as large amounts of aerobic exercise reduce the oestrogen level. However, don't stop altogether, as everyone needs a certain amount of exercise each day (see page 263).

Exposure to light – Go out in bright light for at least 20 minutes a day to encourage your pituitary to produce normal amounts of ovary-stimulating hormones.

Avoid taking non-essential antibiotics – Antibiotics kill most of the bowel bacteria that enable oestrogen to recirculate from the bowel into the bloodstream.

Tests and investigations

These depend on your symptoms, since oestrogen deficiency can be associated with so many gynae problems (see page 295).

Medical treatment

This is chosen according to the gynae problem you have. For example, for a dry vagina after the menopause your doctor may recommend an oestrogen-containing vaginal cream (see page 176).

need to see a doctor?

Yes, if home treatments don't help, if your symptoms are severe or worsening, or if you suspect a gynae cancer.

your action plan

✔ **Vital**
- Dietary changes
- Healthy weight maintenance
- No smoking
- Exercise
- Exposure to light ·

✔ **Could be vital**
- Avoiding non-essential antibiotics

possible gynae or gynae-related causes of some other symptoms

Back pain
- ●●● **Most likely** – prolapse, osteoporosis, stress
- ●● **Less likely** – fibroids, pelvic inflammatory disease
- ● **Possible** – ovary or womb cancer

Aching joints and/or stiff, weak aching muscles
- ●●● **Most likely** – premenstrual syndrome
- ●● **Less likely** – fibromyalgia, chronic fatigue syndrome
- ● **Possible** – sexually transmitted infection, pelvic inflammatory disease, breast infection, under or overactive thyroid

Loss of height
- ● **Possible** – osteoporosis

Abdominal swelling (including bloating)
- ●●● **Most likely** – pregnancy, irritable bowel, obesity, wind
- ●● **Less likely** – premenstrual syndrome, oestrogen dominance
- ● **Possible** – fibroids, ovary cyst, ovary cancer

Weight loss
- ●●● **Most likely** – anorexia
- ● **Possible** – overactive thyroid, any advanced gynae cancer

continued overleaf

Poor appetite

- **Possible** – any advanced gynae cancer, certain drugs

Unusual hunger (plus craving for sweet things)

- **Most likely** – premenstrual syndrome, polycystic ovary syndrome, early pregnancy
- **Possible** – overactive thyroid

Nausea

- **Most likely** – painful period, the Pill, pregnancy
- **Less likely** – pelvic inflammatory disease
- **Possible** – fibroid (twisted), any advanced gynae cancer, anti-cancer chemotherapy

Diarrhoea

- **Most likely** – painful period, irritable bowel
- **Less likely** – endometriosis
- **Possible** – overactive thyroid, gluten sensitivity, ovary cancer

Constipation

- **Most likely** – fibroids, pregnancy, underactive thyroid, irritable bowel
- **Possible** – ovary or womb cancer

Feeling of incomplete emptying of bowels

- **Possible** – fibroids, prolapse, irritable bowel

Painful to open bowels

- **Possible** – episiotomy scar, endometriosis, pelvic inflammatory disease, constipation after gynae surgery

Fear of opening bowels

- **Possible** – prolapse, episiotomy scar, recent gynae surgery

Fluid retention

- **Possible** – premenstrual syndrome, the Pill, certain drugs

Depression

- **Most likely** – premenstrual syndrome
- **Possible** – oestrogen deficiency, gluten sensitivity (which is more common in women than in men), serious gynae illness – especially cancer

Fatigue

● ● ● **Most likely** – premenstrual syndrome

● ● **Less likely** – oestrogen deficiency, anaemia, underactive thyroid, overactive thyroid, chronic fatigue syndrome, fibromyalgia

● **Possible** – any painful condition, any advanced gynae cancer, certain cancer therapies

Headaches and migraine

● ● ● **Most likely** – premenstrual syndrome; unusual sensitivity to pre-menstrual hormone changes or the Pill, stress

● ● **Less likely** – pelvic inflammatory disease; chronic fatigue syndrome (which is more common in women than in men)

● **Possible** – prolactin-producing pituitary tumour

Acne

● ● ● **Most likely** – falling premenstrual oestrogen level, oversensitivity to normal testosterone level, progestogen-only Pill, polycystic ovary syndrome

● ● **Less likely** – high testosterone level, oestrogen deficiency, high humidity, stress

● **Possible** – certain drugs

Unusual hairiness

● ● ● **Most likely** – polycystic ovary syndrome

● **Possible** – oestrogen deficiency, anorexia, certain drugs, androgen-producing ovary or adrenal tumour

Breathlessness

● **Possible** – ovary cancer

Thinning hair on temples and crown

● ● ● **Most likely** – polycystic ovary syndrome

Fever

● ● ● **Most likely** – sexually transmitted infection

● ● **Less likely** – pelvic inflammatory disease

● **Possible** – fibroid (twisted)

periods and menstrual cycles

Most of us have trouble with our periods at some point. Indeed, period pain is so widespread that we might almost consider it normal, and period problems in general, including heavy periods, are the commonest cause of referral to gynaecologists. This section looks at period pain and heavy periods, as well as irregular, scanty or absent periods and bleeding between periods. We will also consider mid-cycle pain, premenstrual syndrome and another common disorder – endometriosis.

period pain

About seven in 10 women who live a 'Westernised' lifestyle sometimes experience period pain low in their abdomen or in their thighs or lower back. It's most common in the teens (although periods are unlikely to be painful until ovulation begins) and early 20s and tends to ease with age, after a first baby and once the menstrual flow increases as a period gets under way.

The pain makes some women feel sick and faint and may also be associated with diarrhoea. At a cellular level it results from increased levels of anti-diuretic hormone, which discourages urine production and oxytocin (both from the pituitary), noradrenaline (from nerves and adrenal glands) and endothelins, nitric oxide and certain prostaglandins (from the womb muscle).

There are two sorts of pain. The more common (spasmodic dysmenorrhoea) takes the form of repeated cramps, similar to labour contractions, starting at the beginning of the period and lasting on average for 12-24 hours. These result from prostaglandins reducing the blood flow in the womb muscle as it contracts to dislodge the womb lining, and from the cervix gradually opening enough to allow the menstrual flow to escape.

The other sort of pain (congestive dysmenorrhoea) is a dull, aching, 'heavy' or 'dragging' sensation that usually starts in the second half of the menstrual cycle and worsens as a period starts. This is caused by fluid retention and by pelvic congestion due to a build-up of blood in the pelvic veins. Some women have both sorts of pain.

Several factors encourage or worsen period pain, including a poor diet. Overweight women often experience more period pain, although this may be attributable to an unhealthy diet rather than excess weight. Other possibilities are a 'coil', fibroids, pelvic inflammatory disease, ovary cysts, and endometriosis in the womb (adenomyosis) – which may be to blame in up to three in five women and causes pain throughout a period. Chemicals inhaled from smoking or passive smoking are another possible culprit. Fibromyalgia (see page 148) encourages period pain too.

what to do yourself

All the time

Healthy weight maintenance – Try to keep to a weight that's appropriate to your height.

Stress management – Find effective ways of dealing with stress.

Dietary changes – Eat a healthy diet, especially in the week before a period, with plenty of foods rich in omega-3 and monounsaturated fatty acids, calcium, magnesium, zinc and vitamins B, C and E. This helps to balance prostaglandin levels and prevent womb cramps. When in pain, try adding a generous amount of parsley to your food, as parsley stimulates the menstrual flow. Consume less refined carbohydrate, fat, alcohol and caffeine-containing drinks, especially in the week before a period. Some women say that meat makes period pain worse, so it might be worth cutting down on this in the week before. Try drinking cumin-seed tea.

Before the pain

Food supplements – Try taking magnesium, calcium and zinc in the week before you expect your period and vitamin E in the two days before.

During the pain

Heat and hydrotherapy – Relax for at least 20 minutes in hot bath water deep enough to submerge your tummy. Alternatively, place a covered hot-water bottle over your lower tummy or tuck a hot pack in your pants.

Exercise – Pelvic rocking (see page 266) and deep breathing may help the pain. If you're capable, exercise may help by boosting your body's levels of endorphins (natural painkillers and mood enhancers).

symptom sorter

Gynae or gynae-related causes of painful periods

● ● ● **Most likely** – disturbed balance of certain hormones, neurotransmitters and/or prostaglandins, poor diet, overweight, coil, smoking, bingeing, stress, fluid retention

● ● **Less likely** – pelvic congestion, fibroids, pelvic inflammatory disease, ovary cysts

● **Possible** – endometriosis in the womb

Massage – Try a 'butterfly' massage – very rapid and light fingertips strokes over your lower spine, as this can help to make pain more bearable (see TENS, below).

Aromatherapy – Help relieve tension and pain by giving yourself an aromatic abdominal massage (lubricating with two drops each of geranium, cypress and rose oils in two teaspoons of carrier oil). Or place an aromatic compress – made with two drops each of clary sage and frankincense oils – over your lower tummy. Or add to your bath water a total of 6-8 drops of these or other oils (such as frankincense, juniper berry, marjoram and rosemary). Note the advice on page 288 regarding the use of aromatherapy oils.

Acupressure – Place your thumb tip four finger-widths above your inner ankle, just behind your large lower leg-bone, and press for two minutes with a small rotatory movement. There's no proof that this works, but it won't hurt to try.

Over-the-counter remedies – Take a non-steroidal anti-inflammatory (NSAID) painkiller such as aspirin or ibuprofen as soon as possible, to help counteract the effects of prostaglandins.

Herbal remedies – Alternate a cup of cramp bark tea with one of calendula or ginger tea every two hours. Lemon balm, fennel, feverfew, and sage teas can be useful too. Or take a twice-daily teaspoon of herbal tincture for two or three days before your period is due, then, when the pain begins, a two-hourly dose. Choose from black cohosh, dong quai, motherwort, mugwort (for dull pain), raspberry leaf, vervain, pulsatilla, *Vitex agnus castus*, and wild yam, or take a dose from two or three tinctures together. *Vitex agnus castus* can be particularly helpful for congestive period pain. Note the advice on page 277 regarding the use of herbal remedies.

Mind techniques – Relax, because tense muscles make pain harder to bear. If life is particularly stressful, search for more effective ways of managing stress (see page 266).

Orgasm – Some women find an orgasm helps, perhaps by decreasing pelvic congestion and encouraging bleeding to begin.

TENS (trans-cutaneous electrical nerve stimulation) – A TENS machine provides electrical stimulation via electrodes stuck to the back and can prevent pain messages from travelling to the spinal cord and brain.

Magnetic or e-m therapy – Devices that produce a magnetic or electromagnetic field, placed beneath your underwear or attached to it, over your lower tummy, are said to help, possibly by increasing the circulation to the womb and so dissipating the build-up of lactic acid produced by its contracting muscle fibres. (See the Helplist, page 315.)

Tests and investigations

You may need a pelvic examination and some women need an ultrasound scan. If you have unfamiliar, uncontrollable, or worsening pain, or have a 'coil', your doctor may take swabs from your cervix to check for pelvic inflammatory disease. Some women need an examination under anaesthetic and a hysteroscopy or laparoscopy, to check for conditions such as endometriosis in the womb's wall, or a twisted fibroid.

> **need to see a doctor?**
>
> See your doctor if the pains persist month after month, worsen, or become unacceptable or you think something else may be wrong.

Medical treatment

Your doctor may prescribe a stronger NSAID painkiller, such as mefenamic acid, naproxen, or rofecoxib, as this works in up to nine in 10 women. If it doesn't, or you also need contraception, consider taking the combined Pill (effective in up to eight or nine women in 10), or taking a progestogen for 20 days a month.

your action plan

✔ Vital

- Healthy weight maintenance
- Stress management
- Exercise

✔ Could be vital

- Heat and hydrotherapy
- Dietary changes
- Over-the-counter remedies
- Medical treatment

(✔) Optional

- Food supplements
- Massage
- Aromatherapy
- Acupressure
- Herbal remedies
- Mind techniques
- Orgasm
- TENS

mid-cycle pain

In some women this often accompanies ovulation, and one possible cause is the rapid increase in size – from 10 to 20mm (⅜-⅝in) in 48 hours – of the main egg follicle as it ripens and stretches the ovary's outer membrane. Another possibility is the release into the pelvic cavity, along with the egg at ovulation, of a tiny amount of irritating blood. These two causes of mid-cycle pain are temporary and nearly always only mildly uncomfortable.

Mid-cycle pain can also result from endometriosis (see page 119).

what to do yourself

If the pain is anything other than mild:

Relax – Try deep-breathing exercises, and rest, if necessary.

Heat and hydrotherapy – Try easing the pain with a warm bath, or hot-water bottle.

Take painkillers – Choose an over-the-counter painkiller such as aspirin or another non-steroidal anti-inflammatory drug, or paracetamol.

Take your mind off the pain – Distract yourself with interesting activities.

Tests and investigations

You may need tests for endometriosis if your symptoms suggest this and are bad enough to warrant medical involvement.

need to see a doctor?

Yes, if the pain is bad (especially if it interferes with your everyday life) or if you have other symptoms.

Medical treatment

Your doctor may prescribe stronger painkillers or treat troublesome endometriosis.

symptom sorter

Gynae or gynae-related causes of mid-cycle pain

● ● ● **Most likely** – ovulation

● ● **Less likely** – endometriosis

your action plan

✔ **Could be vital**

- Relax
- Heat and hydrotherapy
- Painkillers
- Medical treatment

heavy periods

One woman in three says her periods are sometimes either heavy or prolonged enough to disrupt her lifestyle. The formal definition of a heavy period (menorrhagia) is one with a total blood loss of over 80ml (3fl oz or about 5 tablespoons). Studies in which all pads or tampons used in one period were weighed before and after use showed that only one woman in 10 loses this much. However, even a loss of just 60ml each month encourages anaemia.

It's easy to believe that normal periods are heavy because even a little menstrual loss can look substantial and it can be difficult for the individual woman to know what's 'normal'. As a result some women, who mistakenly believe they have heavy periods, receive unnecessary medical treatment that may have side effects.

Measuring the loss is impracticable, but your periods are probably heavy if you:

- use an unusually large number of pads and tampons per period (many more than the average of 22). This may not be an accurate gauge, however, as different women use varying numbers of pads and/or tampons through personal preference or habit

  - have to use two pads at once or change your tampon every hour or two

  - often 'flood', have large clots, or overflow

  - also have unexplained anaemia

Heavy periods may be associated with regular (ovulatory) cycles, or irregular (anovulatory) cycles but in one in two women no cause is established.

Dysfunctional uterine bleeding (DUB)

Heavy or prolonged periods for which no cause is found are referred to as 'dysfunctional' uterine bleeding (DUB). One in five women with heavy or prolapsed periods has DUB. Studies show that one woman in five with DUB doesn't ovulate, so whatever trigger is stopping her ovulation is probably making her periods heavy too. The many possible triggers include stress, depression, infection, other illness, an imbalance of hormones or neurotransmitters, underweight, too much exercise, too little exposure to light and smoking. Failure to ovulate leads to a luteal defect, which means no corpus luteum (see page 21) and therefore a low progesterone level and corresponding 'oestrogen dominance' in the second half of the cycle. Anovulatory cycles (ones in which ovulation does not occur) are often irregular too. Heavy, irregular or abnormally frequent bleeding in a woman's mid to late 40s, is often associated with increasingly irregular ovulation due to her impending menopause.

Other causes of heavy or prolonged periods

- Iron-deficiency anaemia: for while this can result from heavy periods, it can also encourage them, setting up a vicious circle. Indeed, for women living a Westernised lifestyle, heavy periods are the commonest cause of iron-deficiency anaemia.

- Heavy periods are more likely if you have poor diet, with too high an intake of omega-6 fatty acids and not enough omega-3s; this decreases the production of those prostaglandins that help to maintain normal blood-vessel elasticity.

• Bleeding can be excessive because something prevents fibrin (a clotting substance in blood) from working properly.

• An inherited bleeding disorder (such as von Willebrand's disease) encourages bleeding.

• Heavy periods can also result from fibroids, womb polyps, a womb infection (see 'Pelvic inflammatory disease', page 187), inflammation from a recently inserted 'coil', and endometriosis in the wall of the womb.

• Stress and certain drugs.

• Some women blame food sensitivity.

• Over one in two women with an underactive thyroid have heavy periods.

• Smoking worsens heavy bleeding as certain chemicals inhaled from smoke encourage arteries in the womb to bleed for longer than normal.

• Lupus or womb cancer is occasionally to blame.

Note, a 'heavy period' can sometimes, in fact, be a miscarriage.

what to do yourself

No smoking – Smoking makes blood vessels unhealthy and less elastic.

Exercise – Regular brisk exercise promotes healthy blood vessels and hormone levels, both of which can ease heavy bleeding.

Discourage oestrogen dominance – see page 89.

Other dietary changes – Eat more foods rich in calcium, iron, magnesium, zinc, beta-carotene, vitamin C, flavonoid plant pigments, and omega-3 fatty acids, and less of those containing omega-6 fatty acids (see pages 256-260). Try including more cinnamon, said to ease heavy bleeding. Also, try liquidising citrus fruits to give a thick and delicious juice rich in vitamin C and flavonoids. Thyme is another traditional remedy.

Avoid caffeine-containing drinks with meals, as caffeine reduces iron absorption.

Stress management – If you're over-stressed, find more effective stress-management strategies (see pages 266-273). Certainly stress can disrupt menstrual cycles via its effects on the hypothalamus and pituitary.

Identify suspected food sensitivity (see page 261).

symptom sorter

Gynae or gynae-related causes of heavy periods

- ●●● **Most likely** – normal loss, dysfunctional uterine bleeding, oestrogen dominance, 'stress', anaemia, poor diet, coil, smoking, overweight, bingeing, approaching menopause
- ●● **Less likely** – fibroids, endometriosis in the womb, pelvic inflammatory disease
- ● **Possible** – underactive thyroid, food sensitivity, lupus, clotting or bleeding disorder, certain drugs, womb cancer

Aromatherapy – Give yourself a relaxing daily tummy massage, using two drops each of geranium, cypress and rose oils in two teaspoons of sweet almond oil, or put six drops of any of these oils in your bath water. Frankincense, rosemary and fennel oils may also be useful. (Note the advice on page 288, when using oils.)

Food supplements – Consider taking a multivitamin and mineral supplement, but only if you aren't eating properly or feel stressed or unwell.

Herbal remedies – It's best to get personal advice from a medical herbalist, but *Vitex agnus castus* may help to reduce oestrogen dominance. Beth root is an astringent herb and the one most often recommended for heavy periods with no obvious cause; alternatives include ginseng, goldenseal, greater periwinkle, horsetail, and – especially for teenagers – cranesbill, lady's mantle shepherd's purse and yarrow. A uterine tonic herb is a useful addition; examples include black cohosh, dong quai, false unicorn root, raspberry leaf, and squaw vine. Feverfew contains substances that help rebalance prostaglandins by acting as prostaglandin synthetase inhibitors.

(Note the advice on using herbal remedies on page 277.)

Tests and investigations

You'll need a pelvic examination and a blood test for anaemia. If drug treatment (see below) doesn't work, you may need blood tests for thyroid and (especially for teenagers) bleeding disorders. Other options are a transvaginal ultrasound womb scan. If bleeding persists, you may need an endometrial (womb-lining) biopsy, or a hysteroscopy and womb-lining biopsy. These investigations should show whether you have fibroids or polyps, for example.

Medical treatment

Your doctor will treat any identified cause. If the cause isn't obvious and self-help hasn't worked then, if your cycle is regular (which means you're almost certainly ovulating), non-hormone treatments will probably work. In contrast, if your cycle is irregular, you may need hormones. It's important to control the heavy

need to see a doctor?

See your doctor if you don't know why your periods are heavy, if you experience other symptoms or sudden heavy bleeding, if you are worried, if you bleed after the menopause or if home treatments don't work within six months. It's wise to see a gynaecologist if you are over 40 or have other gynae problems or if drugs don't work.

bleeding that's associated with anovulatory cycles, since this shrinks the associated thickening of the womb lining that could, at worst and if continued for a long time, encourage womb cancer.

Your doctor will probably start by recommending a non-hormonal drug such as tranexamic acid, to be taken only during your period. This 'antifibrinolytic' agent helps when blood isn't clotting properly, and halves blood loss in four in five women. Try it for three months; if it helps, you can continue as long as you like. Another possibility is mefenamic acid, a non-steroidal anti-inflammatory drug (NSAID) that can rebalance a disturbed prostaglandin balance. You take it only during a period, and it's worth trying it for three months, or longer if it helps. It reduces heavy bleeding by up to 40 per cent in three in five women, and can be especially useful if your periods are painful, or if heavy periods are due to a coil you want to keep in.

If you would like your treatment to provide contraception, there are four possible drug therapies (and they are particularly appropriate for an oestrogen-dominant hormone imbalance that you can't overcome with lifestyle changes):

- A progestogen-releasing intra-uterine system is the most effective, reducing blood loss by 95 per cent in over nine in 10 women.

- The combined Pill is a useful alternative, halving blood loss in four in five women and regularising periods. If necessary, you can take mefenamic acid as well. If you are nearing your menopause, you can stay on the combined Pill until 51, then try coming off it for three months to see if you've had your menopause.

107

- Progesterone vaginal gel, from day 15 to day 25.
- Progestogens taken for 21 days in each cycle (from days 5 to 25) reduced blood loss by 87 per cent in one study but many volunteers stopped because of the side effects.

If drugs don't work, your doctor may recommend endometrial ablation to remove your womb lining. Hysterectomy, though obviously effective, should be a last resort. One UK study found that less well educated women were more likely to have a hysterectomy than to use drugs for heavy periods (and other period problems). Always go on asking questions until you feel confident you are in a position to make an informed choice.

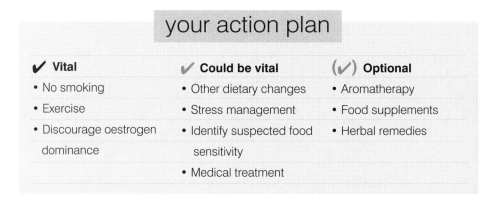

your action plan

✔ Vital	✔ Could be vital	(✔) Optional
• No smoking	• Other dietary changes	• Aromatherapy
• Exercise	• Stress management	• Food supplements
• Discourage oestrogen dominance	• Identify suspected food sensitivity	• Herbal remedies
	• Medical treatment	

irregular, scanty or absent periods

Irregular periods

These often result from irregular or absent ovulation. This is because ovulation is one of the main factors that make periods regular, since menstruation nearly always occurs 14 days afterwards. Irregular ovulation can be perfectly normal for several years after a girl's first period. The first few periods after childbirth are often 'anovulatory' (without ovulation) too, especially if you breastfeed fully and with no long gaps. Sometimes early pregnancy or miscarriage makes a woman think her periods are irregular. And bleeding between periods can make you think you're having an unexpected period. Women who live or work closely together may also develop irregular periods for several cycles as the 'invisible' scent of natural substances called pheromones produced by their armpits and scalp affects their brain and encourages their cycles to synchronise.

Regular ovulation and periods depend on a reasonably good balance of sex hormones from the hypothalamus, pituitary and ovaries. But many factors can disrupt this and cause oestrogen dominance or deficiency. They include stress, depression, excitement, rapid weight loss, being very underweight, bingeing and/or being overweight and too much exercise. Irregular periods often occur for several cycles after stopping the Pill, since the natural hormone balance – and therefore regular ovulation – can take time to re-establish itself. Sex hormone disruption can also be associated with short winter days, which raise the level of melatonin in the body, or frequent long-haul air travel across time zones which disrupts the body clock and causes jet lag.

If you don't ovulate, you have no corpus luteum to produce progesterone, and this 'luteal defect' means you're likely to have oestrogen dominance in the 'second half' of your menstrual cycle (from when you might have expected ovulation up to your period). This can delay a period, make it heavy (see Dysfunctional uterine bleeding, page 104) and cause spotting between periods. It also causes prolonged stimulation of the womb lining in the second half of the cycle by oestrogen 'unopposed' by progesterone. This can lead to overgrowth of the womb lining (endometrial hyperplasia). Continued abnormal oestrogenic stimulation can eventually encourage womb cancer.

If your period generally comes fewer than 11 days after ovulation – in which case you are said to have a 'short luteal phase' – you may have a low progesterone level due to a poorly functioning corpus luteum.

Other causes of irregular periods include

* vitamin B deficiency

* diabetes

* anaemia

* an over- or underactive thyroid

* taking the Pill (especially the progestogen-only 'mini' Pill) or stopping any type of Pill

* blood-pressure medication.

Bleeding between periods (for example from fibroids, polyps, certain ovarian cysts, pelvic inflammatory disease, or cervix, ovary or womb cancer) may mimic irregular periods (see page 113).

Scanty periods, and reversible cessation of periods in premenopausal women

Nine in 10 women with scanty periods have polycystic ovary syndrome, as do up to three in 10 women who have absent periods and are not pregnant or breastfeeding.

A sudden weight loss of 10kg (22lb) or more can stop periods. Sometimes periods fail to return for some months after stopping the Pill. A high prolactin level (see 'Nipple itching and/or discharge, page 70) is found in one in five women with no periods and one in 50 with scanty periods and leads to milk production. Over-zealous removal of the womb lining during an operation called endometrial resection (ablation) can reduce the volume of periods (or stop them permanently). Long-term tamoxifen therapy or gonadotrophin-releasing-hormone analogues for breast cancer, for example, can stop periods. A permanent menopause that's premature or early (see page 220) is also sometimes responsible.

Periods have never started

If a teenager's periods haven't started by 15, the odds are all is well and she's simply a late starter. However, the doctor may need to rule out an anatomical defect in her womb or vagina if she is otherwise physically well developed or, if not, a problem with her endocrine glands, sex chromosomes and/or ovaries.

what to do yourself

Discourage oestrogen dominance and deficiency (see pages 89 and 93).

Also:

Stress management (see page 266) – This is particularly important in teenagers and in women coming up to their menopause, because their hormone balance is less robust, so stress is more likely to disrupt sex-hormone control by the hypothalamus and pituitary.

symptom sorter

Gynae or gynae-related causes of irregular, scanty or absent periods

● ● ● **Most likely** – normal after puberty or childbirth and before menopause; pregnancy; dysfunctional uterine bleeding; the Pill; stopping the Pill; polycystic ovary syndrome; oestrogen dominance; oestrogen deficiency.

● ● **Less likely** – weight loss (including anorexia), bingeing, overweight, too much exercise, 'stress', depression, excitement, short winter days, long-haul air travel across time zones, fibroids

● **Possible** – pheromonal synchronisation, vitamin-B deficiency, diabetes, anaemia, overactive or underactive thyroid, gluten sensitivity, pelvic inflammatory disease, premature menopause, high prolactin level, blood-pressure medication, womb cancer

Other dietary changes (besides those for oestrogen dominance or deficiency, and stress management – page 266) – Eat more foods rich in vitamin B (to counter stress) and vitamin E (to aid hormone production).

Exposure to light – Bright light encourages regular ovulation via its effects on the pineal and hypothalamus. If an ovulation monitor or hormone tests reveal that you are ovulating irregularly, or not at all, you need to spend more time each day in bright outdoor light. Also, consider using a light visor or box in the morning or evening, and doing a six-month trial of sleeping at night with a 100-watt light switched on from days 14-17 of your cycle. It's noteworthy that some chicken farmers – whose livelihood depends on chickens ovulating – supply 24-hour light in chicken sheds to encourage egg production.

Food supplements – Consider taking vitamins B6 and E, evening primrose oil, and plant oestrogens.

Aromatherapy – Put two drops each of rose, geranium and lavender oils in your bath to encourage relaxation and hormone balance, or add to two teaspoons of sweet almond oil for an abdominal massage. Other useful oils include juniper berry, marjoram, rose, fennel, and clary sage. Please note the advice on page 288.

Herbal remedies – It's best to get personal advice from a medical herbalist, but if hormone tests reveal you are ovulating but have a low progesterone level in the second half of your cycle, your options might include a course of *Vitex agnus castus* and/or beth root, starting on the first day of a period. *Vitex* is most likely to be useful if your cycle has a short luteal phase, one with fewer than 14 days between ovulation and your period) or if your cycles are very irregular. If you aren't ovulating, false unicorn root or dong quai may help. Both *agnus castus* and false unicorn root can be useful for unexplained irregularity. If you are nearing your menopause and finding irregular periods a nuisance, black cohosh is probably best. Note the advice given on using herbal remedies, page 277.)

Tests and investigations

Hormone tests may be necessary. If you have irregular periods you may, for example, need tests to measure your levels of luteinising and follicle stimulating hormones: a raised level of both suggests that your ovaries aren't responding, while low or normal levels suggest that

need to see a doctor?

See your doctor if you feel unwell or worried; if you are experiencing fertility problems, bleed after sex, between periods or after the menopause; if you are 16 or 17 and haven't yet had a period or if home remedies don't help within three to four months.

something is affecting your hypothalamus or pituitary. The need for other tests and investigations depends on your symptoms and anything the doctor finds on examination. Sometimes a womb biopsy is necessary.

Medical treatment

Drug treatments include the progestogen-only ('mini') Pill for one to three months; or a course of clomiphene to stimulate ovulation.

your action plan

✔ **Vital**
- Discourage oestrogen dominance or deficiency (pages 89 and 93)
- Dietary changes
- Exposure to bright light
- Effective stress management

✔ **Could be vital**
- Medical treatment

(✔) **Optional**
- Food supplements
- Aromatherapy
- Herbal remedies

bleeding between periods

This can mimic irregular periods. In some women it happens after sex, and light mid-cycle bleeding can also be associated with the normal hormone changes around ovulation.

On the other hand, failure to ovulate can cause bleeding that appears to be between periods but is actually due to irregular periods – or 'dysfunctional uterine bleeding' (see 'Heavy periods', page 103). This is most likely in the teens and the few years before the menopause, when ovulation is more likely to be erratic or absent. In teenagers this is because the hormonal regulation of menstrual cycles can take time to become established, while in older women it's because their low and falling number of eggs discourages regular ovulation.

Other factors that can lead to dysfunctional uterine bleeding by preventing the hypothalamus from balancing sex hormones include:

• abnormal body weight or too much physical activity

• too little exposure to light

• stress

• a thyroid or adrenal gland disorder

Without ovulation there's no corpus luteum, so there's a low level of progesterone in the second half of the cycle. This means the womb lining is stimulated by oestrogen 'unopposed' by progesterone – resulting in an oestrogen-dominant hormone imbalance. This makes various parts of the womb lining break down at different times, leading to spotting of blood between periods.

Other things that can cause bleeding, sometimes just spotting, between periods, include:

• too low a dose of oestrogen in the combined Pill

• the progestogen-only Pill

• one or two missed Pills

• contraceptive hormone injections

• fibroids, polyps in the womb or cervix, ovary cysts, ovary cancer, inflamed cervix, and womb infection

symptom sorter

Gynae or gynae-related causes of bleeding between periods

●●● **Most likely** – can be normal at ovulation, overweight, underweight, too much exercise, too little exposure to light, stress, too low a dose of oestrogen in the combined Pill, progestogen-only Pill, missed Pill, contraceptive hormone injections. Bleeding between periods is often confused with miscarriage or dysfunctional uterine bleeding.

●● **Less likely** – oestrogen dominance, cervical erosion, inflamed cervix, womb infection, atrophic vulvo-vaginitis

● **Possible** – injury from fingernails or sex toy; underactive thyroid; fibroids; womb or cervix polyp; ovary cyst; ovary, cervix or womb cancer; adrenal disorder

symptom sorter

Gynae or gynae-related causes of bleeding during or after sex

●●● **Most likely** – cervical erosion, inflamed cervix

●● **Less likely** – sexually transmitted infection

● **Possible** – recent cervix procedure, fibroid (stuck in cervix), womb or cervix polyp, cervix cancer

• cervical erosion and atrophic vulvo-vaginitis (see 'Dry vagina and vulva, page 173).

• Cervix or womb cancer – the main concern.

what to do yourself

Use home treatments to treat the cause, where possible, but only after a medical check.

Tests and investigations

These depend on your age, history and any findings on examination. For example, you may be advised to have a cervical smear or a trans-vaginal ultrasound scan to assess your womb lining and rule out cancer of the womb. If the scan shows that your womb lining is more than 4mm (⅙in) thick, you may be advised to have a womb-lining biopsy or a hysteroscopy

Medical treatment

If indeed this is necessary, it is chosen according to the cause.

need to see a doctor?

Yes, because you can't usually tell by yourself whether bleeding between periods is normal or not. One exception is if you know that you always bleed when you ovulate, and you've already had a medical check. Others are if your periods have only recently started or if you've recently begun taking the progestogen-only ('mini') Pill or had an intrauterine contraceptive system inserted.

your action plan

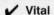 **Vital**
- Medical check to find the cause

✔ **Could be vital**
- Home and medical treatments appropriate to the cause

premenstrual syndrome

Many women notice a particular pattern of physical and emotional changes from 10 days before a period to a day or two after. Some changes, such as increased creativity and energy, are welcome. Others are unwanted or even incapacitating – in which case a woman is said to have premenstrual syndrome (PMS).

PMS can make you feel depressed, irritable, tense, tired, dizzy, faint or forgetful. It can cause sleep problems and mood swings, unusual hunger with cravings for sweet foods in particular. You may retain fluid, leading to weight gain, headaches, bloating and swollen breasts, ankles and fingers. Other possibilities are painful joints or muscles and palpitations (awareness of your heart throbbing). The good news is that while many women experience some of these symptoms, few experience them all.

The cause of PMS remains unclear, but the most likely explanation is that it's due to changes in levels of neurotransmitters such as serotonin and GABA (gamma-amino butyric acid), resulting from oversensitivity to the changing balance of progesterone and oestrogen. During the few days before a period, for example, our serotonin level is at its lowest and the body may still be producing withdrawal symptoms following the fall in endorphin levels after their surge at ovulation. Some researchers believe PMS results from a disturbance of the brain's 'body clock', which helps to regulate the production rhythm of various neurotransmitters and other natural body chemicals.

PMS occurs only in ovulatory cycles and is more likely after coming off the Pill or having a first baby and in the 30s and 40s. It affects up to three in four women at some time and up to 8 per cent of these may have it severely or even be temporarily disabled.

what to do yourself

Keep a diary of periods and symptoms – this will help you to establish whether your symptoms follow a pattern associated with your cycle.

Dietary changes – In the two weeks before a period, avoid letting yourself become very hungry. Eat small, regular meals and favour a healthy diet with plenty of foods rich in calcium, chromium, iron, magnesium, zinc, vitamins B, C and E, beta-carotene and plant oestrogens (see pages 256-260). These help to keep your womb, ovaries, blood, and hormone and neurotransmitter levels healthy. Eat more foods rich in omega-3 fatty acids and less of those rich in omega-6s to encourage healthy hormone levels. Foods rich in the amino acid tryptophan may help but only if low in protein (such as bananas, cauliflower, potatoes, nuts, dates, pumpkin seeds, wholegrain foods) and not if eaten with protein-rich foods. This is because tryptophan must be relatively free from competition with other amino acids in the blood if it's to enter the brain.

Watch out too for bad pre-menstrual dietary habits. Feeling more tired or irritable than usual, for example, could make you reach for fatty, calorie-laden snacks. Also, cut out added salt (to help prevent fluid retention) and reduce your intake of alcohol, caffeine-containing drinks and refined carbohydrates such as sugar.

Healthy weight maintenance – Both excess weight gain and slimming on a crash or fad diet encourage PMS.

Exercise – Take regular, moderate exercise, especially in the two weeks before a period, even if you don't feel like it, because it encourages a healthy hormone balance, reduces stress and raises levels of natural 'feel-good' chemicals such as endorphins (see page 263).

Stress management – Relax and cosset yourself more, especially in the week before your period; you might, for example, give yourself a treat each day. Also, practise prioritising and saying 'no' when necessary.

Get creative – Use the premenstrual week for creative activities calling for emotional expression, such as writing, painting, decorating your home, and wearing clothes in colours that symbolise your feelings.

Exposure to bright light – Get more bright daylight each day. Two hours of bright light in the early evening may help to rebalance any disturbance in neurotransmitters too. This can be achieved by going outside if it's still bright, or using a light box or light visor.

Flashing light – Wearing a mask that flashes red lights for 15 minutes a day for two weeks before their period has been shown to help three in four women (see also page 291 and Helplist, page 315).

Hydrotherapy – Relaxing in a warm bath – perhaps with music playing, a book to read, or just time to daydream – may ease tension.

Acupressure – Put the tips of your thumb and forefinger on either side of a finger of your other hand, at the level of the base of its nail. Press together gently but firmly for a few seconds. Repeat on each finger, then swap hands. This is said to help lift a low mood.

Massage and aromatherapy – Aid relaxation by massaging your legs, arms and tummy, using two drops each of lavender and neroli, and either chamomile or clary sage oils added to two teaspoons of sweet almond or other carrier oil. Or ask someone for a full-body or shoulder massage.

Add to your daily bath three drops each of any two of the following – rose, geranium, neroli and lavender oils – to help relax you and balance your hormone levels. Geranium and rosemary oil may also help to counteract fluid retention while rose oil can be useful for depression and stress.

(Note the advice given on page 288 when using aromatherapy oils.)

Food supplements – try a multivitamin and mineral supplement for a few months. Some studies suggest vitamin B6 helps, but more than 200mg a day can cause side effects. A supplement of plant oestrogens helps some women, as does evening primrose oil.

Herbal remedies – Skullcap and *Anemone pulsatilla* can help, as can yam cream (apply a teaspoon over thighs or abdomen twice daily in the two weeks before a period). Or consider taking a hormone-balancing herb (see page 277) each morning for up to six months. German research found *agnus castus* helped one in two women, whereas a dummy remedy helped only one in four. Swedish research suggests that an extract of rye and certain other grass pollens can reduce weight gain, irritability and depression associated with PMS, possibly because antioxidants (such as flavonoids and superoxide dismutase) in these pollens help the blood vessels to keep the body's fluid balance steady. The pollen extracts are treated to ensure a minimal risk of an allergic reaction, so anyone who suffers from a pollen allergy should be able to take them without any problems.

(Note the advice on page 277 when using herbal remedies.)

Tests and investigations

You may need blood tests to rule out anaemia and thyroid disorders, both of which can mimic PMS.

need to see a doctor?

Yes, if home treatments don't work and your symptoms are unacceptable.

Medical treatment

Mild diuretics can help to counteract fluid retention by increasing urine production: cautions, interactions with other drugs and side effects vary for each drug, so check them with your doctor or pharmacist.

Anti-depressant drugs called SSRIs (selective serotonin reuptake inhibitors) boost the availability of serotonin and can be an effective first-line treatment for severe PMS, according to 15 well-conducted trials. You take them either continuously or in the second half of your cycle but side effects such as nausea, vomiting, 'indigestion', abdominal pain, diarrhoea, constipation, anorexia with

your action plan

✔ **Vital**	✔ **Could be vital**	(✔) **Optional**
• Dietary changes	• Medical treatment	• Acupressure
• Healthy weight	• Creativity	• Massage and
maintenance	• Flashing light	aromatherapy
• Exercise	• Hydrotherapy	• Food supplements
• Stress management		• Herbal remedies
• Exposure to bright light		

weight loss and hypersensitivity reactions are fairly common. Other possibilities include a dry mouth, anxiety, headache, insomnia, drowsiness, tremor, dizziness, weakness, hallucinations, convulsions, milky nipple discharge, sexual dysfunction, sweating, mania, movement disorders and bruising.

There's no good evidence of benefit from the combined Pill, progestogens, or progesterone. Gonadotrophin-releasing hormones (such as danazol), prescribed by gynaecologists, are effective for severe PMS, perhaps because they reduce the mid-cycle rises in the body's own gonadotrophin-releasing hormones; however, their side effects (see page 302) may make them unacceptable.

endometriosis

This name, from 'endometrium', meaning womb lining, and 'osis', meaning caused by, is appropriate because endometriosis is associated with patches of cells identical to those in the womb lining but growing in the wrong place – outside the womb. These patches grow and bleed each month, like those in the womb, because they're under the influence of menstrual hormones; they affect up to one in five women of menstruating age in westernised countries and may occur almost anywhere. However, they are most likely to be on the ovaries, cervix, bladder, urine passage (urethra), bowel, kidneys, gallbladder or elsewhere in the abdomen or pelvic cavity or in the womb's wall (where they're called adenomyosis). Very rarely they occur in the lungs, pancreas, gums, joints, muscles, or even in the nose, eye or ear.

Some women are unaware that they have endometriosis, while in others it causes pelvic or abdominal pain that can be severe. One woman in three with endometriosis has fertility problems caused by patches on her ovaries and/or fallopian tubes and up to one in three women with fertility problems also has endometriosis.

The pain in this condition results mostly from blood formed by the patches during a period making adjacent tissue inflamed. If endometriosis affects the bowel it encourages irritable bowel syndrome and bleeding in the bowel. The inflammation can produce strands of scar tissue called adhesions that can make organs stick together. Depending on their location, inflammation, adhesions or scarring can make it painful to pass water, open bowels or have sex. Some women have cystitis-type symptoms and blood in their urine just during a period.

In some women the pain is continuous, in others it occurs only around ovulation. It readily mimics the pain associated with pelvic inflammatory disease. One study found that in one in four women pain improved spontaneously within a year and in two in four it became worse. The pain usually disappears during and for some years after pregnancy and after the menopause.

About three in five women with endometriosis develop patches on their ovaries that turn into cysts. These look like blood blisters because they fill with blood during each period. Often they break and release their contents into the pelvic cavity, causing pain and inflammation. These cysts can enlarge and, if a large cyst ruptures, it can cause pain so severe that the woman goes into shock and needs emergency surgery. If cysts go on growing, pain is more likely, blood accumulates and older blood darkens, making cysts look dark brown ('chocolate cysts'). Despite all this, the cysts usually subside without treatment.

The cause of endometriosis is an enigma, although there are many suggestions, which is why it's sometimes called 'the disease of theories':

• It can run in families

• It's more common if you have your first baby over 30

• One study found that women who'd ever taken the Pill had double the risk

• It could be due to autoimmune damage (damage by the body's own, normally protective, antibodies). Women with chronic fatigue syndrome, fibromyalgia, an underactive thyroid or allergies are more likely to have endometriosis.

• 'Retrograde menstruation', in which some of the menstrual flow (which contains womb-lining cells) enters the abdominal cavity via the fallopian tubes, could be a cause. However, this is common in all women and normally the stray cells disappear, so something would have to happen to allow the cells to 'take root' and cause endometriosis. (Also, the retrograde menstruation theory wouldn't account for endometriosis in the nose and lungs.)

Trouble is more likely for women who have an oestrogen-dominant hormone imbalance, especially one with a low progesterone level in the second half of their menstrual cycle, meaning oestrogen is 'unopposed' (see 'Irregular periods', and 'Bleeding between periods, pages 108 and 113'). Endometriosis is also more common in women who have used tampons for more than 14 years.

what to do yourself

Reduce oestrogen dominance – see page 89.

Dietary changes – Eat a healthy diet, as this helps to counteract inflammation and relieve stress. In particular, eat plenty of foods rich in omega-3 fatty acids, beta-carotene, vitamins B, C and E, magnesium, selenium, zinc, flavonoids, salicylates (in most fruit, vegetables, nuts), plant oestrogens and fibre and have some low glycaemic-index (GI) foods (see page 26) at each meal.

Avoid rapid increases in blood sugar by eating high-GI foods only in small amounts. Eating less meat, eggs and dairy food may reduce inflammation by promoting a better balance of prostaglandins. Try cutting down on coffee, as there's an unproven suggestion that too much may encourage endometriosis.

Stress management – Feeling stressed can worsen pain and inflammation, so use more effective stress-management strategies if necessary (see page 266).

Consider having your first baby earlier rather than later – Endometriosis tends to worsen with time, so may encourage fertility problems as you get older.

Alternative sanitary protection – Consider using only sanitary towels, especially at the height of your period, since a saturated tampon may not absorb the menstrual flow fast enough to allow good drainage via the vagina, possibly encouraging blood to be forced out through the fallopian tubes.

'Butterfly' massage – Do a light, rapid, fingertip massage (a 'butterfly' massage) over your lower spine to help reduce pain.

Aromatherapy massage – A gentle tummy massage, using three drops of lavender oil in two teaspoons of sweet almond oil, may relieve pain.

Hydrotherapy – Relaxing in a warm bath may help you to manage pain.

Herbal remedies – Drink a cup of ginger tea twice a day to help relieve inflammation. Besides this, it's best to consult a medical herbalist for personalised advice but herbs that may help include paeony (counteracts oestrogen dominance and relieves pain), *Vitex agnus castus* or false unicorn root (reduces oestrogen dominance), dandelion root (boosts the liver's breakdown of oestrogen), dong quai (reduces pain), and feverfew (relieves pain from inflammation). (Note the advice on page 277)

Tests and investigations

The only way of confirming endometriosis is for a gynaecologist to do a laparoscopy and see the patches somewhere in the abdomen or pelvic cavity.

Medical treatment

Mild pain may improve with non-steroidal anti-inflammatory painkillers, such as naproxen, that inhibit the production of inflammatory prostaglandins. Hormones help to control pain in up to four in five women by reducing or preventing bleeding; they do this by counteracting oestrogen or in other ways. However, they don't treat the cause, often have side effects and are not suitable if you're trying to get pregnant. Also, the pain returns in one in two women within five years of stopping. The options are equally effective, and the choice is usually based on side effects and costs. They include:

need to see a doctor?

Your doctor can help to ascertain whether you have endometriosis. If your doctor suspects endometriosis, and your symptoms are troublesome, it's wise to see a gynaecologist. Many women and their doctors don't recognise what's wrong for years, leading to unnecessary delay in getting specialist help.

• The low-dose combined Pill – which has relatively rare and, nearly always, only minor side effects. 'Tricycling' is often recommended – taking the Pill continuously for nine weeks, then waiting a week – when you'll have a 'period'.

• A progestogen-releasing intrauterine system; in one survey this greatly helped seven in 10 severely affected women.

• Progestogens – taken continuously and often prescribed initially for nine months. This is more likely than the progestogen-releasing intrauterine system to trigger side effects.

• GnRH (gonadotropin-releasing hormone, or gonadorelin) analogues, such as buserelin and goserelin – continued use helps by lowering the oestrogen level but the side effects may be unacceptable.

• Danazol and gestrinone – continued use helps by lowering the oestrogen level but the side effects may be unacceptable (although this is less likely than with gonadorelin).

One unofficial survey of the members of an endometriosis self-help group found drugs relieved symptoms in only 10-15 per cent, though this figure may be skewed since many of the women in such a group would have joined *because* they hadn't found relief from other treatments.

Other options

Depending on their location, a laparoscopy may enable some patches to be destroyed – for instance with heat from a laser beam or with a jet of helium gas. A chocolate cyst on the ovary may need surgical removal if a woman is infertile and the cyst is preventing successful fertility treatment. In a few cases pain may be controlled only by removal of the womb and ovaries.

your action plan

✔ **Vital**	✔ **Could be vital**	(✔) **Optional**
• Dietary changes	• Alternative sanitary	• Butterfly massage
• Reduce any oestrogen	protection	• Aromatherapy
dominance (page 89)	• Medical treatment	massage
• Stress management	• Herbal remedies	• Hydrotherapy
	• Consider having a first	
	baby earlier	

fertility

Many of us tend to think of fertility as a right and imagine that we can control it with contraception or have a baby when we choose. However, not everyone is capable of having a baby at all, let alone to order. The good news is that lifestyle changes, plus, most important, aiming to start your family while you're relatively young, can make a big difference to fertility. Medical intervention, if necessary, can also enable some women to conceive.

fertility problems

Conceiving may take longer than you think, even if you are both fertile. 90 per cent of fertile couples having regular sex take up to a year to start a baby, while 5 per cent take up to two years. Among couples who do not conceive within a year or two, research shows that 40 per cent of fertility problems stem from the woman, 30 per cent from the man and 30 per cent are unexplained. More than one factor may be involved; each partner may contribute to the problem and some men and women are infertile only with certain partners. The most common causes of female infertility are failure to ovulate and damage to the fallopian tubes. The most common cause in men is 'dysfunctional' sperm.

Female causes

Polycystic ovary syndrome (PCOS)

This is the most common 'cause' of female fertility problems, since many women who have it don't ovulate. However, it is the factors responsible for PCOS, rather than PCOS itself, that are to blame.

Age

Many young working women today delay their first baby until they are over 30, but the longer they leave it, the more likely they are to be disappointed.

fertility and age

- The decline in female fertility begins at 27, and it goes down ever faster after 35.

- As a woman ages her egg supply dwindles and when only about 25,000 remain (at age 37, on average) they dwindle twice as fast. The older a woman is the fewer eggs she has and the less fertile she becomes.

- Ageing eggs lose quality and are more likely to have sustained damage to one or more of their genes or whole chromosomes. This encourages infertility, miscarriage, and congenital disorders. The chance of a woman over 42 having a baby naturally is under 10 per cent. This is partly because by then nine in 10 of her eggs will have developed a chromosomal abnormality such as that in Down's syndrome. In contrast, only one in 10 chromosomal abnormalities in unborn babies results from an abnormal sperm.

- Peak fertility for the most fertile of couples has been said to be no more than 33 per cent in any one menstrual cycle. However, a recent European study found the chance of conceiving in any cycle to be 50 per cent at 19-26 years old, 40 per cent at 27-34, and under 30 per cent at 35-39.

- A woman aged 35 takes twice as long to conceive as one aged 25.

- Each month a 38-year-old has only a quarter of the chance of a woman under 30 of conceiving a healthy baby.

- In the USA half of all 35-45 year-old women have difficulty conceiving or carrying a baby to term.

- Women in their early 30s who have fertility treatment using their own eggs have a 30 per cent chance (or more) of giving birth to a live baby but women of 43 or older have only a 3 per cent chance.

It may be that, one day, young women will be able to opt to pursue a full time career and have children when they are older by freezing egg-containing ovarian tissue or embryos. However, the likelihood of conception using previously frozen ovarian tissue or embryos is currently very small, with only just over 12 per cent of women in the UK who have had a previously frozen embryo implanted, for example, giving birth to a live baby.

The 'G-Test' – in which the degree of ovarian oestrogen production following a nasal spray of gonadotrophins indicates the number and quality of remaining eggs – helps to predict whether fertility is likely to continue for another two years.

Blocked or damaged fallopian tubes

This is most often due to chlamydia infection (now said to be responsible for one in three cases of infertility), other infection, pelvic inflammatory disease or adhesions (strands of tissue due to inflammation or scarring) following endometriosis or pelvic surgery. Having an ectopic pregnancy in which a baby settles in a fallopian tube leads to its destruction.

Other causes

Many factors besides PCOS and age can prevent ovulation and you should always suspect this if your periods are irregular and heavy or light. If you don't ovulate, you have no corpus luteum, so the progesterone level is very low in the couple of weeks or so before your period – that is, in what should have been the luteal phase of your cycle. This is one sort of 'luteal defect'. Another type of luteal defect happens when you are ovulating but your corpus luteum isn't working properly and so isn't producing enough progesterone in the second half of your cycle. This means you are likely to menstruate fewer then 11 days after ovulation. A poorly functioning corpus luteum can encourage very early miscarriage; indeed, an 'infertile' woman may actually be miscarrying repeatedly and very early, without realising that she has conceived. (Among the other causes of repeated early miscarriage is the existence of antibodies that trigger clots in the placenta.)

Several lifestyle factors can encourage infertility by disturbing a woman's hormone balance and, perhaps, preventing ovulation, including lack of exposure to bright daylight in winter, being over- or underweight, eating a poor diet, smoking, being continually over-stressed and exercising excessively.

Obviously, not having sex around ovulation can be responsible for infertility. Sometimes the mucus produced by the cervix is hostile to sperms. Drugs can cause infertility too; possibilities include certain 'anti-psychotics' (for example, for schizophrenia) and selective serotonin reuptake inhibitors (for example, for depression) – which lower a woman's oestrogen and progesterone levels and raise her prolactin level. A raised prolactin level due to other causes (see 'Nipple itching and/or discharge, page 70) can also cause infertility. Sometimes infertility is the only sign of sensitivity to gluten (a protein in wheat, barley and rye); other possible signs of gluten sensitivity include a swollen abdomen, stomach ache, diarrhoea, weight loss, illness due to nutrient deficiencies, mouth ulcers, depression, irregular periods, osteoporosis and bowel cancer (see page 250).

Some studies, though not all, suggest that using a 'coil' can be to blame. One investigation found that having a coil for six years or more gave only a one in four chance of conceiving within a year of its removal. Women with a coil were also more likely to have an ectopic pregnancy (one outside the womb). The longer you use a coil, the greater the chances are of pelvic infection; if such an infection spreads to the fallopian tubes and is either undiagnosed or unsuccessfully treated, the tubes may be too badly damaged to enable an egg to pass.

A woman who has radiotherapy of an ovary or surgery to remove an ovary, before the age of 30, is likely to experience her menopause seven years early, so it's wise not to wait too long to try for a baby. If surgery for an ovarian cyst is required, it's worth asking if the surgeon can remove only the cyst not the ovary. Women undergoing any cancer treatment also have a higher risk of infertility.

Male causes

Up to 10 per cent of men are infertile, most often because of sperm dysfunction – meaning the sperms are structurally abnormal, don't move properly, don't live long enough or can't swim through the mucus in the woman's cervix. Male fertility declines from the age of 35 as the sperm count and quality decline. A man may be less fertile if he is overweight, eats a poor diet, is sensitive to gluten (see above), drinks too much alcohol, smokes or is stressed. Exposure to environmental oestrogens is also under suspicion. Too little bright daylight in winter reduces sperm production. Some men have a low sperm count because they make antibodies that destroy their sperm; others because varicose veins in their scrotum heat one or both testes. Finally, men who have treatment for cancer may risk infertility and may want to consider having sperm frozen beforehand.

what to do yourself

Aim to identify and avoid, modify or treat possible risk factors.

Many couples can do several things to improve their chance of conception. Suggestions for both of you are included here, as some couples won't know which partner needs to take action.

For both of you:

Stop smoking – or, at least, cut down, as smoking encourages early miscarriage.

Give up or limit alcohol – as it can encourage early miscarriage.

Dietary changes – Eat a healthy diet, as this provides vitamins B, C and E, folic acid, selenium and zinc to nourish sperms and eggs and help sperms swim. (Even a slight lack of zinc can reduce a man's testosterone, sex drive and sperm count.) Eat more omega-3 fatty acid-rich food and less omega-6-rich food, to aid healthy hormone production and immunity. Favour organic produce, since a small proportion of salads, vegetables and fruits fails tests for safe levels of pesticide residues and certain pesticides can lower the sperm count and encourage miscarriage. One study suggests that an amino acid called arginine may improve fertility, possibly by improving the circulation to the ovaries. Arginine-rich foods include nuts, seeds, cereal grains, corn, rice and chocolate. Also eat less lysine-rich food (fish, shellfish, eggs, meat, eggs, milk, yogurt, beans – especially bean sprouts, potatoes) as this reduces your response to arginine.

Healthy weight maintenance – Losing excess weight can increase male and female fertility. It can also make medical fertility treatment more successful. For example, if an overweight woman isn't ovulating and has polycystic ovary syndrome, losing weight improves her chances of conceiving. And all overweight women having medical fertility treatment have a 75 per cent better chance of conceiving if they lose weight.

In contrast, if you're so underweight that you don't ovulate, gaining weight could make you fertile again. Aim for your 'body mass index' (BMI, see 'Overweight, page 241) to be at least 20, preferably more. If it's 18 or 19 you'll have periods, but won't ovulate, and if it's below 18, you won't even have periods.

Manage stress wisely – Any stress can prevent ovulation and lower the sperm count. And using home methods of encouraging fertility (such as taking your temperature each morning so that you can be sure to have sex when your temperature rises in mid-cycle) could make you anxious or disappointed, reduce sexual desire and arousal and even spoil your relationship. Effective stress-management strategies are therefore very important.

Exposure to light – Go outside in bright daylight for at least 30 minutes each day to promote normal hormone balance and encourage normal ovulation and sperm formation. If you live a long way from the equator (such as in northern Europe, or in Canada), consider wearing a light visor or using a light box in the morning or evening.

Identify any suspected food sensitivity – see page 261.

Occupational protection – Take recommended precautions if you work with industrial or agricultural chemicals. Female health workers and airline-crew exposed to ionising radiation should consult their occupational physician. It could be advisable to arrange a job with the lower exposure limit usually assigned only for pregnant women. Textile industry workers and dental-surgery assistants may benefit from a prolonged break or change of job. Consider changing jobs if your current job is particularly stressful.

Food supplements – Women should consider a mineral and vitamin supplement specially formulated for the peri-conceptual time, and men should consider a general multi-mineral and vitamin supplement.

Also, for women:

Predict ovulation – The average woman with an average-length cycle ovulates on day 14 (day 1 being the first day of her period). So she is most fertile on days 10-15 inclusive and particularly days 13-15. However, the length of normal, regular, ovulatory cycles varies in different women from 24-32 days. As there are nearly always 14 days between ovulation and the period, a woman with a short cycle will ovulate earlier (for example, with a 24-day cycle, on day 10), and a woman with a long one, later (for example, with a 32-day cycle, on day 18).

An egg must be fertilised within 24-36 hours of ovulation. However, this doesn't mean conception can occur only if you have sex then, because sperms usually survive up to 72 hours in the vagina, womb and tubes, and when the cervical mucus is 'fertile' (see below) some can live as long as five days. The timing of sex that's most likely to be successful is from 72 hours before ovulation to 36 hours after.

The week before you expect ovulation, aim to have sex each morning, because most women ovulate in the afternoon and it helps if sperms are waiting. Researchers claim it's preferable for fertility to have sex only once a day. Aim to have an orgasm as the resulting changes in the volume and chemistry of your cervical mucus help sperms swim to the egg and an orgasm makes the womb 'suck up' sperms. Gravity may further help sperms if you lie on your back, with your hips raised on a pillow, during sex and for 20 minutes after.

The following methods will help you to predict or detect ovulation and give you the best chance of having sex at the 'right' time:

Menstrual diary – Keep a diary of your periods to help predict your most fertile time each month. Nature isn't always predictable, though, and some women ovulate unexpectedly, like rabbits, in response to sex.

Check vaginal moisture – 'Fertile' mucus produced around ovulation encourages sperm to travel to the womb and tubes as it's much more plentiful than 'infertile' mucus, and much thinner, clearer, and more slippery and stretchy. If stretched between finger and thumb it forms a very long string. Ovulation occurs within 24 hours (sometimes 48) of peak mucus production.

Use an ovulation-prediction kit (from pharmacies) – A few days before you expect ovulation, a colour change in a paper stick dipped in your urine shows whether you are making enough luteinising hormone to enable conception.

Use an electronic ovulation-predictor monitor (such as the Persona, from pharmacies in the UK) – This stores and collates information about hormone levels over several cycles, then signals with a coloured light the likelihood that you are fertile. For example, with one monitor when you insert a urine-moistened paper stick into it, a red light shines if you are fertile, yellow if you might be, and green if you're not.

Use a microscope – Two or three days before ovulation, the oestrogen and progesterone levels in saliva are such that you can see a distinctive fern-like pattern of crystals on a slide smeared with saliva and viewed through a microscope. If you see this pattern, using a testing kit, you know that ovulation is likely to occur very soon.

Body temperature – Consider taking your temperature before you get up each morning and watch for the rise of around 0.4°F (0.1°C) that occurs just after ovulation – though this isn't very accurate.

Discourage oestrogen dominance or deficiency (see pages 89 and 93).

Herbal remedies – It's best to get personal advice from a medical herbalist. Consider, for example, taking *Vitex agnus castus* for six months and for longer (12–18 months) if your hormone levels improve. In one study, 39 out of 45 'infertile' women taking this herb became pregnant. False unicorn root is another traditionally used herb. If your periods are irregular and perhaps heavy, the herbal remedies discussed for these conditions (see page 111) may help trigger regular ovulation. Note the advice on page 277 when using herbal remedies.

Also, for men:

Avoid beer – Its plant oestrogens and certain other ingredients can depress the sperm count.

Keep your scrotum cool – A man who drives for long hours should consider a break or change of job until his partner conceives, as a prolonged seated position heats the testes and can depress sperm production. Men whose jobs involve heat-exposure (e.g.welders) might also find a break helps. Men were once advised to boost fertility by favouring loose – and therefore cooler – boxer shorts rather than tight underpants and by avoiding tight jeans. However, research has demonstrated that this makes no difference to semen quality.

Herbal remedies – Consider taking ginseng, which can increase sperm production and help to regulate hormone levels and astragalus, which can encourage sperms to move more efficiently.

Tests and investigations

Besides a physical examination, several other things may help.

For women. A blood test for progesterone on day 21 of your cycle indicates whether you have ovulated (and if repeated in several cycles, whether you are ovulating regularly), or whether you have a low progesterone level and therefore a luteal defect (see page 21). If your cycle is irregular, it's worth doing the progesterone test seven days before the earliest you might expect a period, then every five days until your period starts. Tests of follicle-stimulating hormone (FSH) and luteinising hormone (LH) are also useful; they are done between days two and five of your cycle if you are having periods or at random if you have irregular periods or none. A raised FSH suggests the store of eggs in your ovaries may be running low; a raised LH (plus normal FSH) suggests you have polycystic ovary syndrome. Alternatively, repeated trans-vaginal ultrasound scans detect whether you are ovulating by looking for a ripening follicle and thickening womb lining.

need to see a doctor?

One in six couples in the UK seeks medical help with fertility. Until recently, most experts recommended medical help in the form of IVF and other 'assisted reproduction' techniques (see 'Medical treatment', below) for over-30s who hadn't conceived during a year of regular, frequent sex and for over-35s who hadn't conceived during six months of the same. However, it has recently been suggested by European experts that over-30s with no obvious reason for infertility should wait for 18-24 months before getting this sort of help, simply because – given enough time – many of them conceive naturally.

A blood test showing high levels of chlamydia antibodies indicates a high chance of damaged fallopian tubes.

Other possible tests include blood tests for prolactin (helpful if you have irregular or absent periods or are producing milk though you haven't been pregnant or had a baby; if the result is high this could indicate a prolactin-producing growth in the brain); sex-hormone binding globulin and testosterone (which could indicate polycystic ovary syndrome) and thyroid stimulating hormone. Also potentially useful for some women are an ultrasound scan; laparoscopy, X-ray of womb and tubes following insertion of radio-opaque dye ('hysterosalpingogram'), hysteroscopy, womb-lining biopsy and a blood test for chromosome analysis.

For men. A sperm count; a normal count is 30-120 million per millilitre of semen, with 60 per cent normally formed and 60 per cent active after two hours. If the count is abnormal the test is repeated four to six weeks later and sperm antibody and strength tests done. Blood tests can indicate hormone levels and provide chromosomes for analysis; some men need a testis biopsy.

For both. A blood test for gluten sensitivity and, if positive, an intestinal biopsy (done via a swallowed viewing tube – an endoscope).

Medical treatment

Always ask about the likely success rate of any treatment and the risk of problems before accepting it.

For women with fertility problems

Depending on what is causing your problem, the possibilities include:

- Vaginal progesterone gel, taken cyclically, to counteract a low progesterone level in women who are ovulating but have a luteal defect.

- Progestogens, taken cyclically, to counteract a low progesterone level in women who are ovulating but have a luteal defect.

- Drugs to stimulate ovulation. Clomiphene latches on to oestrogen receptors in the hypothalamus, preventing a woman's own, stronger, oestrogen from latching on and discouraging gonadotrophin production. Follicle-stimulating hormone, luteinising hormone and human chorionic gonadotrophin can also stimulate ovulation. Bromocriptine can reduce an inexplicably high prolactin level. (Note that certain hormone therapies can encourage breast and ovary cancer, so have a breast check before starting treatment, and ensure that your doctor is aware of any family history of either cancer.)

- Microsurgery to try to clear blocked fallopian tubes.

- Removal of a fibroid.

- Destruction of patches of endometriosis.

- IVF-ET – *in vitro* fertilisation (IVF, '*in vitro*' meaning in a test tube) plus embryo transfer. This involves the surgical removal of eggs, fertilising them in a dish with some of your partner's sperm and putting the embryo(s) into your womb via your vagina. In the UK, doctors put back only two (occasionally three) embryos. The chance of success from this and other IVF techniques (including ICSI, see 'For men with fertility problems' below) is 29 per cent in women of all ages, 33 per cent in women under 38. These are excellent figures if you compare them with those in fertile couples (see 'Fertility and age', page 125). One in 100 children born in developed countries are conceived by IVF.

symptom sorter

Gynae or gynae-related causes of fertility problems

● ● ● **Most likely** – failure to ovulate, blocked fallopian tubes, polycystic ovary syndrome, ageing, oestrogen dominance, oestrogen deficiency, lack of bright daylight, obesity, bingeing, underweight, poor timing of sex, sex too frequent or infrequent, smoking, too much exercise, poor diet, partner factors.

● ● **Less likely** – endometriosis, pelvic inflammatory disease, sexually transmitted infections, over or underactive thyroid.

● **Possible** – gluten sensitivity, fibroids, high prolactin level, certain drugs, cancer treatment.

- Surgical removal of your eggs, their fertilisation with your partner's sperm in a test tube and the placing of the resulting embryo(s) – or 'zygote(s)' – in one of your fallopian tubes. This is called ZIFT, or zygote intra-fallopian transfer.

- Surgical removal of your eggs ('gametes') followed by placing them in one of your fallopian tubes. This is called GIFT, or gamete intra-fallopian transfer.

- Egg donation (donor IVF), which involves eggs being donated by another woman and mixed with your partner's sperms in a test tube, then put in your womb. Donated eggs are usually surplus to the donor's fertility treatment, though can be removed from any fertile woman who's been on ovary-stimulating hormones. The success rate is around 40 per cent.

- Embryo donation – the same can be done with an embryo formed from a donated egg and donated sperm.

- Womb transplants may be possible one day; a donor womb could come from a woman who has had a hysterectomy or the infertile woman's mother or sister. One such operation has already taken place at the time of writing, though it has not enabled a successful pregnancy.

- Researchers are experimenting with ovary tissue transplants. An 'autologous' transplant uses a woman's own ovary tissue that's been surgically removed and deep-frozen before cancer treatment that will destroy her eggs and cause an early menopause. When she decides to try for a baby the stored ovary tissue is inserted beneath the skin of her arm and she takes hormones to stimulate the production of eggs that can be removed for test-tube fertilisation. This experimental technique raises the possibility that some women who do not have cancer may, one day, choose to have ovarian tissue stored so that they can delay pregnancy. Also, as deep-frozen ovarian tissue doesn't age, a post-menopausal transplant could even act as natural HRT. And, theoretically, a woman could choose to become pregnant in her 50s, 60s or beyond, though few would wish to do so!

- The world's first ovary transplant, from one sister to another, has recently been done in China, though at the time of writing no pregnancy has resulted.

- One day it may even be possible to grow a baby in an artificial womb.

For men with fertility problems

The possibilities vary according to the problem:

- For 'dysfunctional' sperms the usual treatment is injection of a single sperm (ejaculated, or removed by needle or biopsy) into a surgically removed egg. This is called intracytoplasmic sperm injection (ICSI); it is a type of IVF and its success rate – 30 per cent – is astonishingly good.

- Placing the man's sperms directly into the woman's womb, usually after hormonal egg stimulation; this IUI (intrauterine insemination) makes pregnancy twice as likely.

- IVF (see above).

- Gonadotrophin therapy (see page 302).

- Surgical removal of sperms from the man's testis or epididymis if his ejaculated semen contains no sperms.

- Surgery for extensive varicose veins in the scrotum (a 'varicocele').

- Insemination of the woman with donated sperm. This is called sperm donation, or DI – donor insemination.

For either of you

It's claimed that the world's first artificially cloned baby has just been born at the time of writing. A 'clone' has genes that are identical to those of its parent and in contrast to naturally occurring identical twins, triplets or more, an artifically cloned baby has only one genetic parent. Artificial cloning is done by inserting genetic material from a body cell (not an egg or a sperm) into an empty egg cell, then applying electrical stimulation. However, scientists are concerned that artificially cloned babies, like artificially cloned animals, may have a high risk of certain age-related diseases. Cloning is illegal in most developed countries and remains, to all intents and purposes, unavailable.

your action plan

For both of you

✔ **Vital**

• No smoking

• Give up or limit alcohol

• Dietary changes

• Healthy weight maintenance

• Stress management

Also, for women

✔ **Could be vital**

• Predict ovulation

• Discourage oestrogen dominance
  or deficiency

Also, for men

✔ **Could be vital**

• Reduce beer intake

• Keep your scrotum cool

• Occupational protection

• Exposure to light

✔ **Could be vital**

• Identify any food sensitivity

• Food supplements

• Medical treatment

(✔) **Optional**

• Herbal remedies

ovaries

Although they are tiny, our ovaries have an enormous impact on our health and lifestyle via their influence on our hormones, periods and fertility. So anything going wrong with them can cause problems with our periods, breasts, fertility, womb, cervix, vagina and vulva. All of these are considered in the relevant sections. Here, however, we will look at cysts on or in the ovaries, and ovary cancer.

ovary cyst

Lumps called cysts, some filled with fluid, some solid, often develop in an ovary. Multiple cysts are more likely before the menopause, single ones after. A 'follicular cyst' develops in the follicles ('pockets') around eggs that have started ripening and is most likely in 20-40 year-old women. In premenopausal women one in two such cysts disappears spontaneously – sometimes in a few days and usually within a month or two, sometimes six. The other most likely type of premenopausal cyst is associated with polycystic ovaries. Less common are luteal cysts, which are formed in the corpus luteum if it fails to disappear, can delay a period and usually go within a few weeks or months and cysts formed by bleeding into patches of endometriosis. Dermoid 'cysts' are solid benign growths resulting from a developmental abnormality and containing hair, teeth or other tissue unrelated to the ovary.

Most cysts are trouble-free, but some produce oestrogens, progesterone, or, rarely, androgens and some cause bleeding between periods, pelvic pain, abdominal pain and fullness, painful sex, frequent urination, weight gain, and swelling of the abdomen. Occasionally a cyst bursts, bleeds, twists on a stalk ('torsion') or becomes infected. Ovary pain is most likely either side of the middle of the abdomen, but if a cyst bleeds or bursts, there may be more generalised abdominal pain.

After the menopause, single cysts are more likely, and around 30 per cent of these disappear spontaneously. Some, though, keep on growing and a few grow extremely large. Occasionally a cancer grows in the wall of a cyst; indeed, one in three ovary cysts that develops after the age of 45 is cancerous.

137

Tests and investigations

If your doctor's examination reveals an enlarged ovary – bigger than 5cm (2in) across – an ultrasound scan will reveal any ovary cyst and show whether it is fluid-filled or solid. (An MRI or magnetic resonance imaging scan or a CAT or computerised axial tomography scan may be done in some countries.) A blood test for CA125 (see Ovary cancer, page 144) will suggest whether it's likely to be cancerous.

need to see a doctor?

If you have one or more of the symptoms outlined above, and they are unexplained, see a doctor to assess the cause and, if you have an ovary cyst, to establish which type they are and whether they need medical treatment. Get medical help urgently if you have a fever or severe abdominal pain, in case an ovary cyst has become infected or twisted.

If a cyst doesn't go within two or three months – or more than a month in a woman over 45 – or if it's troublesome or solid, your doctor may recommend a laparoscopy to view it and, perhaps, drain it, remove it or take a biopsy.

Medical treatment

The Pill may help to prevent certain ovary cysts.

A surgeon may remove a cyst estimated to measure less than 7.6 cm (3in) across during a laparoscopy. One possible drawback to this, though, is that if what's thought to be a benign cyst turns out to be a cancer, operating through a laparoscope may not enable the surgeon to remove it completely, in which case the surgeon will do a laparotomy; an operation under a general anaesthetic in which a cut is made in your lower abdomen. There is also a risk of cancer cells leaking and spreading the cancer as the cyst is removed.

Removal of a larger cyst needs a laparotomy. You'll be back to normal activities within two to four weeks, although sometimes a cyst returns and also, the operation may trigger infection, damage the bowel or bladder or encourage the formation of adhesions – strands of internal scar tissue that sometimes cause problems (see page 184).

Sometimes, the whole ovary has to come out (an operation called oophorectomy). Having only one ovary decreases fertility, so if you need surgery and want to become pregnant in future, ask the surgeon if it's possible to remove only the cyst. If you have an ovary removed before the age of 30 you are likely to have your menopause seven years earlier than you otherwise would. So if you want to get pregnant, it may be wise not to wait too long.

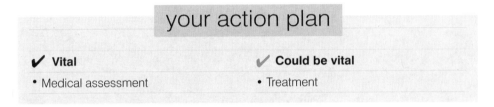

your action plan

✔ **Vital**
• Medical assessment

✔ **Could be vital**
• Treatment

polycystic ovary syndrome

At some time in her life, one in every three or four women develops polycystic ovaries – which means her ovaries become studded with multiple cysts that are bubble-like and up to 8mm (⅜in) across. Normally, several egg follicles start growing in the first half of the menstrual cycle, then one becomes dominant and ruptures to release an egg. But in a woman with polycystic ovaries this mechanism is upset, so none of her follicles becomes dominant.

Up to one in three women with polycystic ovaries has polycystic ovary syndrome (PCOS), which means having ten or more cysts, plus some combination of:

• **Obesity.** Over one in three women with PCOS are overweight or often binge. Production of testosterone and other androgens is raised in overweight women, some of this extra testosterone is converted to oestrogen, and the ovaries and pituitary become 'confused', encouraging egg follicles to become cystic, and disturbing menstrual hormone cycles, ovulation and periods. Interestingly, most women with bulimia have polycystic ovaries.

• **Difficulty conceiving**. Polycystic ovaries – though not necessarily PCOS itself – are present in three in four women who aren't ovulating regularly, four in five who aren't ovulating at all, up to nine in 10 with infrequent periods and over two in five with previously unexplained infertility.

• **Irregular or absent periods**. Up to 60 per cent of women with PCOS have irregular periods and 25 per cent have none at all.

- **Acne.** Around one in three women with persistent acne has PCOS.

- **Excess facial and body hair.** While more than four in five 'hairy' women have PCOS, at least one in two women with PCOS have excess facial or body hair.

- **Thinning of hair on temples and crown.** In one study of 101 women with this 'male-pattern' thinning, 72 had PCOS and thinning was sometimes the only symptom.

PCOS usually begins in the teens or 20s and symptoms often begin after gaining weight suddenly, or stopping the Pill. It can run in families and is the most common hormone disturbance in women. Various lifestyle factors encourage the hormone imbalance often associated with PCOS including stress, obesity and bingeing. In some women with PCOS, their body cells fail to use energy at a higher rate after a meal – a process that normally accounts for 80 per cent of our energy use. PCOS can also be triggered by phenytoin, an anti-epilepsy drug.

The cells of many women with PCOS are relatively insensitive to insulin. This problem is usually associated with a woman being overweight or eating an unhealthy diet with too much high-glycaemic-index (GI) food (see page 140) and not enough low-GI food. Insulin resistance leads to high blood sugar, low cell-sugar levels and, eventually, to a high insulin level. Researchers think this is the key factor in PCOS and one which also increases the risk of diabetes, high blood pressure, and stroke. Being overweight can cause or worsen insulin resistance, though many women with PCOS aren't overweight, so the underlying cause remains unclear. Some women with PCOS and insulin resistance have 'acanthosis nigricans' – rough, darkened, thickened skin in their armpits and groins and on the nape of the neck.

A high insulin level tends to raise the levels in the blood of free testosterone and other androgens. This is probably because it reduces the level of sex hormone binding globulin (which normally mops up a proportion of male hormone molecules – leaving fewer available to exert their influence by latching on to cell receptors). High testosterone encourages acne, male-pattern hair thinning and excess facial or body hair, though the 'high' level found in some women with PCOS is still much lower than that in a man.

There may also be a high level of oestrogen (mostly oestrone, made from androgens in fat cells). However, in spite of this – or perhaps, partly, because of it – the egg follicles don't mature properly and instead become cystic, no one follicle ripens fully and ovulation is often irregular, or stops. This causes irregular, infrequent or absent periods and, perhaps, infertility, though the pituitary gland tries to get the cycle back on track by producing a high level of luteinising hormone. Lack of ovulation causes continued stimulation of the womb lining in the second half of the cycle, which thickens the womb lining and may disrupt womb-lining cells, increasing the risk of womb cancer. If periods are absent the risk is higher, since the womb lining continues to be stimulated yet is never shed.

The menopause in a woman with PCOS is likely to be early.

what to do yourself

Discourage oestrogen dominance (see page 89).

Healthy weight maintenance – Losing excess weight and keeping your new, healthy weight stable make your cells more sensitive to insulin, which is the best way of restoring regular periods and reducing hairiness. Losing weight is also the best way of increasing fertility, since you're unlikely to ovulate if you are obese (which means having a body mass index of over 30, see page 241). Do it with a sensible diet, exercise and stress-management plan.

Other dietary changes – Eat a healthy diet to help balance hormones and protect arteries. Have regular small meals with some low-glycaemic-index (GI) food at each meal. Avoid rapid increases in blood sugar by eating high-GI food only in small amounts, and choosing foods rich in chromium (mushrooms, wholegrain foods, and liver), magnesium, manganese, zinc, fibre, and plant oestrogens. Dietary plant oestrogens may help, as they tend to increase the level in the blood of sex hormone binding globulin – a protein that binds testosterone and thereby reduces its action. Also, consider liquidising and eating a whole orange, (including the peel) each day; researchers say inositol (related to vitamin B) in the peel reduces insulin, testosterone and sugar levels.

Exercise – Help to balance hormone levels and protect arteries with half an hour's brisk daily exercise.

Exposure to light – Go outside in bright daylight for longer than usual each day to help balance hormones. This may be particularly important if you are overweight, often binge on carbohydrates, or suffer from winter depression.

Although any benefits are unproven, it may also be worth using a light box or a light visor in the early morning, or evening.

Acne and excess hair remedies – Over-the-counter acne products may help mild to moderate acne and plucking, depilatory creams, bleaching, shaving, waxing, electrolysis and laser therapy can help to manage unwanted hair.

Herbal remedies – It's best to consult a medical herbalist for personalised advice. False unicorn root contains plant oestrogens that may help to counteract a high oestrogen level without suppressing ovulation. Black cohosh may be particularly helpful if you are stressed. And paeony or *Vitex agnus castus* may help an imbalance of oestrogen and progesterone and/or of luteinising hormone (LH) and follicle stimulating hormone (FSH) and a high level of prolactin or testosterone. Liquorice or sarsarparilla (wild liquorice) is a useful addition to help acne and excess body hair. (Note the advice on page 277 when using herbal remedies.)

Consider acupuncture – There is no proof that this helps but reports indicate that it helps horses, cows, pigs and dogs with PCOS, so it may be worth trying.

Tests and investigations

An ultrasound ovary scan can reveal multiple small cysts with a transvaginal ovary scan being most reliable. However, this isn't necessarily a great help as many women without polycystic ovary *syndrome* as such have polycystic ovaries. If you have irregular periods, a womb scan reveals any abnormal thickening of the womb lining.

Blood tests reveal any disturbance in hormones. The most common test is for LH, and is done in the first five days of the cycle. A raised level (one of over 12 iu/l) suggests PCOS. (The level of FSH is normal in women with PCOS.) Blood tests may also be done for testosterone or prolactin. If you have a high testosterone your doctor may rule out

need to see a doctor?

Your doctor can confirm PCOS and suggest a package of home and medical treatments you need to prevent or control your symptoms. In teenagers it may be difficult to distinguish normally irregular periods plus obesity or other PCOS-type symptoms, from PCOS itself, so a doctor will probably recommend watching and waiting to see what happens. Any woman who has adult acne, or whose hair is falling out for no obvious reason before the menopause, should discuss the possibility of PCOS.

other possible causes – such as an adrenal or thyroid disorder and if you have a high prolactin, your doctor may need to rule out a pituitary tumour. You also need urine and blood tests for diabetes and blood tests for blood fats and cholesterol.

Medical treatment

This depends on your weight, age and plans to have children and is secondary to lifestyle factors such as losing excess weight and eating a healthy diet. If you find irregular periods a problem, or your womb lining is particularly thick (over 15mm or ⅝in), the Pill can help by causing monthly periods and thereby reducing the raised risk of womb cancer associated with a thickened womb lining. It also, of course, provides contraception.

If you are bothered by excess facial and body hair a contraceptive Pill containing cyproterone acetate plus oestrogen, for 21 days a month, usually reduces hair growth by up to a third over six months. It also makes each hair finer, which makes electrolyis easier and skin damage less likely. Cyproterone is a powerful progestogen that inhibits the production of gonadotrophins (follicle stimulating hormone and luteinising hormone), thus reducing androgen production in the ovaries. It also attaches itself to androgen receptors so it blocks the action of androgens. This therapy also produces regular periods and can help insulin resistance and acne (though it's worth trying over-the-counter or prescribed acne treatments first). One problem is this medication could make it more difficult to lose weight and weight loss is often a vital part of successful treatment. Possible side effects include weight gain, nausea, tiredness, low sex drive, breast tenderness, headaches, depression, irritability.

The progestogen-only Pill also reduces excess hair and another possibility is cream containing a hair-growth inhibitor drug called eflornithine.

If your main concern is infertility drug therapy with clomiphene or tamoxifen triggers ovulation in 70-90 per cent of women with PCOS, though only 30-70 per cent will conceive. If this doesn't work your doctor may try FSH, which enables 70-80 per cent to ovulate and 20-40 per cent to conceive. Less common treatments include cauterisation (destruction by heat) of large cysts during laparoscopy and IVF (test tube fertilisation). If a high oestrogen level has led to a high prolactin level you may need treatment with bromocriptine.

Researchers are investigating a drug called metformin that appears to help by making cells more sensitive to insulin. However, a recent study shows it doesn't encourage ovulation in women with fertility problems associated with PCOS.

your action plan

✔ **Vital**
- Healthy weight maintenance
- Dietary changes
- Exercise
- Discourage oestrogen dominance (page 89)
- Stress management
- Exposure to Light

✔ **Could be vital**
- Medical treatment

(✔) **Optional**
- Acne and excess-hair remedies
- Herbal remedies

ovary cancer

Women in the UK have one of the highest risks in the world, and it is the fourth most common cancer in women in the UK and Australia, fifth in the US. Ovary cancer is rare under 40 and most common after the menopause but your risk is reduced if you have ever taken the combined Pill. Indeed, taking the Pill for just three years can halve your risk.

Ovary cancer is sometimes called the silent killer, since its early symptoms may be considered too vague to report to a doctor. This means that up to three times in four it has spread beyond the ovary by the time it's discovered, which is why the average five-year survival for all women with ovary cancer is only 30 per cent. However, 95 per cent of women with early ovary cancer do have symptoms, so it's worth all women taking such symptoms seriously, for if treated early enough, around four out of five women are still alive after five years.

The most common symptoms are slight abdominal discomfort (usually low on one side of the tummy, near the umbilicus, or in the groin) and bloating – which is easily mistaken for middle-age spread. Other possibilities include fatigue, nausea, indigestion, persistent constipation or diarrhoea, weight loss, back pain, pain during sex, increased urination, and vaginal bleeding. Sometimes it's difficult to distinguish the symptoms of ovary cancer from those of irritable bowel syndrome. And sometimes the first sign is when the cancer grows so large you can feel it, or it causes fluid retention in the abdomen, or it pushes up against the diaphragm and causes breathlessness.

The risk rises with age, with around nine in 10 women being over 45. There are several other risk factors, the most important being a history in your close family – as 5-10 per cent of women with ovary cancer have inherited a damaged BRCA1 or BRCA2 gene, which makes this cancer more likely. If your mother has had ovary cancer your risk is six times that of the average woman and if your sister has had it your risk is nearly four times the average. If two close relatives have had it, you have a two in five risk of getting it – which is very high, so it's essential to see a gynaecologist to discuss screening. Sometimes a high risk of both ovary and breast cancers or of both ovary and colon cancers, runs in families.

Another risk factor is repeated hormonal stimulation of the ovary, associated with having a relatively large number of ovulatory menstrual cycles in your life. This means that the later your periods start, the longer you're on the Pill, the more pregnancies you have, the longer you spend breastfeeding and the earlier your menopause, the lower is your risk of ovary cancer. A woman who has never had a child has double the risk.

Repeated use of fertility drugs (such as clomiphene) can encourage ovary cancer. Contrary to older, smaller studies, a major Swedish study reported in 2002 shows that being on HRT may increase the risk.

Drinking too much alcohol on a regular basis encourages ovary cancer. Other factors that remain under suspicion include:

• frequent use of dark hair dye, as certain potential cancer-trigger chemicals ('carcinogens') can pass through the scalp into the blood

• talcum powder and 'feminine deodorants' used on the tummy or vulva, or a sanitary towel, since irritating particles can travel up the vagina and through the fallopian tubes to the ovaries

• mumps viruses

• a high level in the blood of lactose (milk sugar) in women who can't break it down because their gut lacks an enzyme called lactase.

Having your first baby early has a protective effect, as does being on a Pill containing a relatively high dose of progestogen. Like certain other cancers, ovary cancer is less likely in women with allergies; researchers suspect this may be because they make relatively large amounts of immunoglobulin E (IgE) antibodies. These seek out pollens, house-dust mites and other allergens, and it's possible that they also seek out cancer cells and encourage their destruction. So researchers are investigating safe ways of stimulating IgE production.

what to do yourself

To help *prevent* ovary cancer you need to lead a healthy lifestyle and take general anti-cancer measures (see page 84). Aim to minimise controllable risk factors, ensure that you have any recommended screening and always report unexplained symptoms early. Interestingly, research suggests that taking a small dose of aspirin at least three times a week reduces the risk of the commonest type of ovary cancer by about 40 per cent. However, this can't yet be recommended, as there is no proof and aspirin can have side effects.

To help treat cancer lead a healthy lifestyle, take general anti-cancer measures (see 'Gynae' cancers, page 84) and minimise controllable risk factors, as some of these may influence cancer growth.

If your risk is raised because one or more of your close relatives has, or has had, ovary, breast or colon cancer – especially if they had it before 50 – ask about annual screening with transvaginal ultrasound scans and a blood test for CA125. This is a protein that's produced by cancer cells and raised in over four in five women with ovary cancer. However, its level can also be raised by many other factors, including menstruation and pregnancy, and is sometimes normal in a

need to see a doctor?

See a doctor if any of the above symptoms continues for several weeks or is severe or if you are worried. General practitioners in the UK are encouraged to refer all women over 50 with unexplained abdominal symptoms to a cancer-unit gynaecologist for an ovary-cancer check.

woman with ovary cancer. Your doctor may suggest you go on a Pill with a relatively high dose of progestogen.

If your risk is very high, and you don't want children in future, you may want to discuss the option of having both ovaries removed. This virtually prevents the risk of ovary cancer (and also reduces the risk of breast cancer). Research suggests that being sterilised by having your fallopian tubes cut can also reduce a high genetic risk of ovary cancer.

Tests and investigations

Possibilities, if ovary cancer is suspected, include a physical examination, a transvaginal ultrasound scan, a blood test for CA125 and, perhaps, a laparoscopy.

Medical treatment

Treatment is with surgery to remove the ovaries and, perhaps, the womb and cervix. You may need anti-cancer drugs (chemotherapy), other drugs or radio therapy. The two most effective drugs are carboplatin (a platinum compound) and paclitaxel (from Pacific yew tree bark). Researchers are experimenting with the laser destruction of cancer cells (perhaps after sensitising them with light-attracting pigment). If after surgery you are left with one ovary and your womb, you can still have children. However, if you have radiotherapy or surgery to remove one ovary, before 30, your menopause is likely to occur around seven years early and your fertility will probably decline relatively fast before this. So if you want a baby you may not want to wait too long.

your action plan

✔ **Vital**

- Medical treatment
- Minimise controllable risk factors
- Take general anti-cancer measures (see page 84)

womb and cervix

It's wise to use a combination of natural therapies and medical treatments to treat disorders of your womb and cervix, just as it is when you're treating disorders of any other part of your reproductive tract. Here we'll look at what you can do to help prevent and treat fibroids, a prolapsed womb and polyps or cancer of the womb and cervix. Infection of the womb and/or tubes is covered under 'Pelvic inflammatory disease'.

fibroids

These gristly, whitish, slow-growing, non-cancerous growths ('leiomyomas') in the wall of the womb are common in the late 30s and early 40s and found in around one in four over-35s. They contain mostly muscle plus some fibrous tissue, are usually multiple, and sometimes protrude into the womb cavity or abdominal cavity. They can be as small as an orange pip or as large as a melon. They often enlarge in the two weeks before a period and in the years just before the menopause.

One in two women with fibroids finds them troublesome and fibroid symptoms are the most common health concerns taken to a gynaecologist. The larger or more numerous your fibroids, the more likely you are to have symptoms. Possibilities include heavy, prolonged periods, perhaps with clots and anaemia, and occasionally painful or irregular periods or bleeding between periods. A large fibroid may press on the bowel, bladder, or blood vessels, encouraging a feeling of incomplete emptying of the bowel, constipation, frequent and urgent urination, or varicose veins. Fibroids occasionally trigger premenstrual syndrome, low backache with a dragging sensation, painful periods or discomfort during sex. Other possibilities are weight gain, abdominal swelling, fertility problems and recurrent miscarriages.

Fibroids can cause four other rare but important problems:

• A fibroid on a stalk may get stuck in the cervix, causing period pain and bleeding and pain during and after sex. This calls for surgical removal.

• One in 1000 fibroids becomes cancerous.

• A fibroid may twist, cutting off its blood supply and causing a fever, nausea, severe pain and tenderness until it shrivels, becomes impregnated with calcium and forms a harmless 'womb stone'.

• In pregnancy a fibroid can break down and encourage miscarriage.

The good news is that fibroids nearly always shrink after the menopause; however if you take HRT they may not shrink as expected and may even enlarge (although this is unlikely).

An oestrogen/progesterone imbalance can encourage fibroids. Scientists think either of these hormones can 'turn on' genes for various growth factors in the womb, leading to local overgrowth of womb-muscle fibres. Fibroids are more likely in very overweight women because their fat cells manufacture oestrogen and they tend to have relatively high levels of blood sugar and growth hormone. Fibroids grow more quickly in pregnancy but are less likely in women who have had a child. They are two to three times more common, develop earlier and grow larger in black women than in white. It's also possible that pelvic congestion (see page 184) encourages fibroids by obstructing the flow in the blood and lymph vessels. The resulting pressure in the wall of the womb might make it more likely to 'defend itself' by forming lumps.

Also, fibroids can run in families and scientists suspect that this may have a genetic basis.

what to do yourself

Dietary changes – Eat more foods rich in plant oestrogens; beta-carotene, vitamins B (including vitamin-B-like inositol, in fruits, beans, peanuts, chick peas, lentils, vegetables and wholegrain foods), C and E; magnesium; and fibre. Also, eat foods rich in methionine (beans, garlic, lentils, onions and seeds) and choline (beans, peanuts, lentils, chick peas and wholegrain foods): methionine is a sulphur-containing amino acid that helps to prevent fat from building up and, together with inositol and choline, lower the oestrogen level. Eat more food rich in omega-3s and less food rich in omega-6s.

Eat less fat, particularly the saturated variety and less refined carbohydrate (foods made with white flour and added sugar). Some women report improvement if they eat less red meat.

Healthy weight maintenance – Lose excess weight and maintain your new, healthy weight.

Exercise – Take half-an-hour's aerobic exercise each day to boost the womb's circulation and reduce congestion and fluid retention.

Orgasm – It's possible – though unproven – that regular orgasm might help to prevent or shrink fibroids by increasing the pelvic circulation and so reducing any congestion and fluid retention in the womb's wall.

Food supplements – There are suggestions that fibroids may improve in women taking vitamin B complex, vitamin E, methionine, choline, magnesium, and plant oestrogens.

Hydrotherapy, heat and cold – Boost the womb's blood supply with a daily contrast sitz bath (see page 274).

Herbal remedies – It's best to get personalised advice from a medical herbalist, although one possibility is to take two hormone-balancing herbs, *Vitex agnus castus* and false unicorn root, each morning. If, after two months, this hasn't helped, lady's mantle may be useful, as it helps counteract a high oestrogen level and reduce heavy bleeding. Other useful herbs for heavy bleeding include beth root and raspberry leaves. (Note the advice on page 277 when using herbal remedies.)

Tests and investigations

An ultrasound scan or hysteroscopy can reveal fibroids.

Medical treatment

need to see a doctor?

No, if your fibroids were discovered by chance and you are symptom free. Yes, if you don't know what's causing your symptoms or if known fibroids become troublesome.

Options, chosen according to circumstances and needs, include waiting to see if mild symptoms improve with the home remedies. This is especially wise if you are nearing your menopause when fibroids are likely to shrink or if the side effects of treatment are likely to be worse than the symptoms.

- A drug called tranexamic acid can help; this is an antifibrinolytic agent that reduces heavy bleeding by reducing the blood flow. Hormonal alternatives to reduce heavy bleeding include the progestogen-only Pill and the progestogen-releasing intrauterine system (which may even shrink fibroids).

- Small fibroids can be removed along with the womb lining during endometrial resection or ablation, done via a hysteroscope passed through the vagina.

- Larger fibroids can be 'shelled out' (myomectomy) either during keyhole surgery, using a laparoscope passed through the abdominal wall (suitable only for small fibroids on the inside of the womb), or during a laparotomy (open abdominal surgery done via a larger incision under a general anaesthetic). You'll need about three or four weeks to recover after a laparoscopy, four to six weeks after a laparotomy. However, laparoscopy or laparotomy may be suitable only if you have one or two fibroids. Also, there's a risk of infection and of serious bleeding (sometimes so bad that a hysterectomy is needed). Up to 60 per cent of women develop strands of internal scar tissue (adhesions) that could cause pain and other problems. There's a risk the womb may rupture (especially with laparoscopy) and a one in three chance of fibroids regrowing. Both operations can damage the bowel or bladder and reduce fertility.

- A technique still being assessed involves destroying a fibroid with laser light via a hysteroscope under MRI (magnetic resonance imaging) guidance.

- Uterine artery embolisation is a promising option involving an overnight stay in hospital. A doctor threads a thin flexible tube into your groin under local anaesthetic. Under X-ray guidance he or she threads it into one of the womb's two arteries then injects plastic or gelatin-foam particles to block the artery. The resulting reduction in blood supply shrinks the fibroids to, on average, half their size and four in five women then have much less trouble. Trials have shown it to be successful eight or nine times in 10. It is suitable for large and small fibroids and may reduce the need for hysterectomy. Is also has relatively low complication and recurrence rates and is safer than myomectomy. However, it isn't suitable if you plan to have children as it reduces fertility. Possible complications include period-like pains for a couple of months, womb infection leading to hysterectomy, transient lack of periods and early menopause in up to one woman in 20, although mainly in women over 45.

• Another option, if the above procedures are unsuitable or don't work, is a hysterectomy. Fibroids are the leading reason for a hysterectomy in the USA, accounting for nearly one in three such operations. It usually has to be done via an abdominal incision, not through the vagina, because of the large size of a womb containing fibroids large or plentiful enough to require this surgery.

your action plan

✔ **Vital**	✔ **Could be vital**	(✔) **Optional**
• Dietary changes	• Orgasm	• Food supplements
• Healthy weight maintenance	• Medical treatments	• Hydrotherapy, heat and cold
• Exercise		• Herbal remedies

polyps

These are non-cancerous fleshy lumps attached by stalks to the lining of the cervix or womb. Sometimes a womb polyp protrudes into the cervix or vagina or a cervix polyp protrudes into the vagina. They may cause no problems and be discovered only during a medical examination or an investigation such as an ultrasound scan done for some other reason. Alternatively, they may cause light bleeding (possibly just spotting) between periods, perhaps only during or after sex or a medical examination; increased production of moisture and, perhaps, depending on their location, discomfort.

What causes polyps is not known, although they are more likely to develop in women taking tamoxifen for breast cancer. There's no known way of preventing them.

need to see a doctor?

Yes, for an initial diagnosis and to discuss whether or not to have the polyp removed. For while a polyp may never cause you any trouble, its removal might be recommended so as to exclude it as a possible cause of any unexpected vaginal bleeding (between periods or after the menopause), in the future. This could be useful, as bleeding can be a sign of womb cancer.

Medical investigations and treatment

The doctor will probably send you to a gynaecologist for an ultrasound womb scan. If this suggests a womb polyp, you'll probably need a hysteroscopy to diagnose the problem and a biopsy to confirm it isn't a cancer; the polyp can be removed at the same time, especially if it's been causing problems such as bleeding during sex.

A cervical polyp is usually simply removed in a young woman but an older woman may also need a womb biopsy to exclude any other problem.

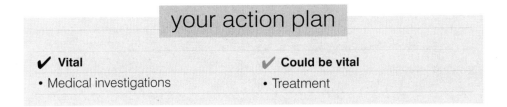

your action plan

✔ **Vital**	✔ **Could be vital**
• Medical investigations	• Treatment

prolapse

Having a prolapse means that your pelvic floor no longer adequately supports your pelvic organs. This occurs when its muscles, ligaments and other tissues have become slack, inelastic and weak and are under stress. The bladder and urethra are most likely to prolapse, followed by the womb, rectum, or urethra alone, in that order.

A prolapse makes you feel as if something is 'coming down' and there may be a lump in your vagina. The sensations usually increase when a woman stands, or increases the pressure in her pelvic cavity by coughing, sneezing, straining to open bowels or lifting a heavy weight. When you lie down, your prolapse may go some or all the way back to its normal position. Some women have backache or a dragging feeling in their pelvic cavity, especially after standing up for some time. Any sort of prolapse can make sex uncomfortable. Having a prolapsed rectum may make opening your bowels difficult because you fear it will make your prolapse come down more. And having a prolapsed bladder can be associated with cystitis-type symptoms of leaking, frequent urination and a burning sensation on passing water. At worst, a prolapse descends enough to pull the vagina's walls inside out like a sock and appear at the vaginal opening.

Many factors can weaken the pelvic floor. They include repeated pregnancies; a long second stage in labour (the stage when you push the baby out of the womb and down the vagina); a forceps delivery, ageing, smoking, a low post-menopausal oestrogen level, being overweight or constipated or having a chronic cough.

what to do yourself

Don't push too early – During childbirth, resist the urge to push until your midwife or doctor gives you the all clear, which is when your cervix is fully opened and has a smooth rim. Otherwise, pushing weakens the pelvic floor and encourages a prolapse later.

Pelvic-floor exercises – Daily pelvic-floor exercises (see page 265) are the most important way of helping prevent a prolapse because they strengthen the pelvic floor. They can alleviate symptoms and prevent a mild prolapse from progressing.

Exercise – Take a daily half hour of brisk 'whole-body' exercise, such as walking, as this improves the pelvic blood flow, which helps to keep pelvic floor muscles strong and elastic

Prevent constipation – Aim to do this by eating a healthy diet, drinking plenty, and taking daily exercise because being constipated and straining to open your bowels can weaken the womb's supports.

No smoking – Stop smoking (or, at least, cut down) to discourage a smoker's cough and chronic bronchitis and – since smoking destroys vitamin C – so you don't rob your pelvic floor muscles and ligaments of the strengthening effects of this vitamin.

Healthy weight maintenance – Aim to maintain a healthy weight, as the weight of excess fat in your abdomen and pelvic cavity could stretch your pelvic floor.

Avoid lifting – Avoid lifting anything heavy, if possible, or lift carefully, holding the weight close to you and keeping your back straight.

need to see a doctor?

Yes, if you are uncomfortable, have cystitis-type symptoms, or your prolapse interferes with your sex life.

Dietary changes – Eat more foods rich in vitamin C, plant pigments and calcium to strengthen muscles and ligaments.

Hydrotherapy – Have a daily contrast sitz bath (see page 275); this helps to boost the pelvic circulation and may improve the condition of your pelvic floor.

Tests and investigations

Your doctor will examine you, and check that your urine isn't infected if you have cystitis-type symptoms. If you need surgery for a prolapse and suffer from leaking, for example, your doctor may recommend that you have bladder volume and urine flow measurements with a view to having surgery for the leaking at the same time.

Medical treatment

A prolapse repair operation can help to support the sagging organ and the type of surgery depends on the type of prolapse. Another option is a hysterectomy plus a repair.

If you are either waiting for surgery, are not fit for surgery or don't want it, your doctor can fit a polythene ring pessary in your vagina to support your prolapse and make you more comfortable; you will need a new ring pessary every three to 12 months. It has been suggested, though not proven, that HRT may help prevent a prolapse from worsening.

your action plan

✔ **Vital**

- Don't push too early in childbirth
- Pelvic-floor exercises
- Exercise
- Prevent constipation
- No smoking

- Healthy weight maintenance
- Avoid lifting
- Dietary changes

(✔) **Optional**

- Hydrotherapy

inflamed cervix

An inflamed cervix – 'cervicitis' – means that something is irritating your cervix and making it inflamed. The inflammation may cause more or less continuous pelvic pain that some women recognise as coming from their cervix. It may also cause pain and, perhaps, bleeding during sex and pain from a tampon or during a medical examination. It can increase the normal production of cervical moisture or, depending on what's responsible, create a discharge that may be brownish or smelly.

The causes include a sexually transmitted infection (most likely chlamydia, but possibly herpes or gonorrhoea) or other infection. Other possibilities are irritation from a cervix polyp or a womb polyp or fibroid protruding into the cervix; a forgotten tampon or diaphragm or repeated rubbing from the penis, fingernails or a sex-toy vibrator. Pre-cancerous or cancerous changes in the cervix can also be responsible, although inflammation is uncommon with these conditions.

what to do yourself

If pain or other symptoms make you suspect this problem, check that you haven't left a tampon or diaphragm in by mistake. If neither of these is the case, you should see your doctor. Once you have a diagnosis you can treat the condition accordingly.

Tests and investigations

Your doctor will probably do a physical examination, check that you've had regular cervical smears (and do one if necessary), rule out other possibilities (such as a cervical 'erosion') and take swabs from the cervix for the laboratory to check for infection.

need to see a doctor?

Yes, unless the problem is a forgotten tampon or diaphragm that you've been able to remove and the symptoms have gone.

Medical treatment

This depends on the cause but if there's an infection, local antibiotics (in the form of a cream or pessary) and, perhaps, oral antibiotics will be necessary.

your action plan

✔ **Vital**

- Medical assessment (if you have ruled out a forgotten tampon or diaphragm)

✔ **Could be vital**

- Appropriate home and medical treatments

cervical 'erosion'

This means that the lining of the passage through the cervix has extended on to the outer part of the cervix (in the vagina). This lining is glandular and more delicate than the normal covering of the outer cervix, so it bleeds easily, for example, with tampons, during sex or when having a cervical smear. Other possible symptoms include pain during sex and an increased vaginal discharge (because the cells produce moisture and are prone to infection).

Cervical 'erosion' is better but less familiarly known as 'ectropion', since there is no actual erosion. It's most common in teenagers, in pregnancy and in women on the Pill. And, as it's stimulated by oestrogen, it is encouraged by anything that leads to oestrogen being 'unopposed' by progesterone in the second half of the cycle (see Irregular periods, page 108, and Bleeding between periods, page 113), by other causes of oestrogen dominance (see page 89) and by the combined Pill, pregnancy and HRT.

what to do yourself

If your erosion began during pregnancy, it's likely to heal itself after pregnancy. Otherwise:

Follow the lifestyle tips that discourage oestrogen dominance (page 91) – These include guidelines on dietary changes, healthy weight maintenance, exercise, exposure to bright light, and avoiding xeno-oestrogens.

Consider coming off the Pill or HRT.

Tests and investigations

Your doctor will look at your cervix through a vaginal speculum, ask if you are up to date with your cervical smears and do one if it's due or there's any doubt about the diagnosis.

Medical treatment

A doctor can destroy the out-of-place cells and so enable normal ones to grow by inserting a speculum and either applying silver nitrate, or using electro-cauterisation with an electrically heated wire, 'cold coagulation' or a laser beam.

need to see a doctor?

Yes, if your symptoms are bothering you or to discuss using alternative contraception or coming off HRT.

your action plan

✔ **Vital**

• Discourage oestrogen dominance (see page 89)

✔ **Could be vital**

• Consider coming off the Pill or HRT

• Medical treatment

abnormal cervix cells/ cervix cancer

One in 100 women in Europe and North America develops cervix (cervical) cancer and it is the most common women's cancer in the developing world, affecting one in 20 in parts of Africa, India and Latin America. Cervix cancer arises where the more fragile mucus-producing cells lining the passage through the cervix meet the tougher cells covering the outer part of the cervix. It can happen at any age but is most common in the early 30s. If not caught early it's often fatal but the good news is that it's much less likely to occur if you have regular cervical smears because these allow any abnormal cells to be observed with more frequent smears, or treated. Abnormal cells are not cancerous but have an increased risk of becoming so and discovering them early prevents most cervix cancers.

Abnormal cells don't usually cause symptoms. Cancer, though, can be associated with bleeding between periods or during and after sex, post-menopausal bleeding, pelvic pain and, perhaps, a bloodstained and smelly vaginal discharge, due to an inflamed vagina. It may also make sex uncomfortable. As it grows, it destroys adjacent tissues and it may eventually cause more widespread damage, or even kill.

Various factors encourage cervix cancer, but the most important by far is persistent human papillomavirus (HPV, or wart virus) infection combined with abnormal cells. This infection is almost always sexually transmitted and makes the cervix more vulnerable to other risk factors. Cervix cancer is rare in women who have never had sex.

HPV infection (see also page 204)

HPV infection is by far the most common sexually transmitted infection, affecting one in three women in their 20s, for example and one in two women at some time in their lives. Although HPV is a wart virus the strains that cause cervix cell abnormalities, or cancer, do not usually cause warts on the cervix (or indeed the vulva). Each new sex partner increases your risk of catching HPV and the more partners your current partner has had, the higher the risk that he will give you HPV. Four out of five young women with HPV shake it off without medical treatment within a year and nine out of 10 within three years but many women become re-infected. If infection persists, the older a woman is, the less likely it is to clear spontaneously. The presence of abnormal cells also means it's less likely to clear. One recent study of women with a high-risk strain of HPV (see below), found that 46 per cent of those with normal cells were infection-free within a year and 100 per cent within four but only 29 per cent of those with mild cell changes were clear within a year and 85 per cent within four.

While short-lived infection doesn't encourage cervix cancer persistent infection, or repeated re-infection does, especially if it's with the same high-risk strain. This could be because the state of the woman's immunity not only tends to prevent her from clearing the infection or resisting re-infection but also makes her more vulnerable to cancer triggers. Such triggers include the Pill and smoking (which stops certain protective cells working properly by 'switching off' the activity of P53 tumour-suppressor gene). The coexistence of *Herpes simplex* viral infection also encourages cancer.

All that being said, only a tiny fraction of women infected with one of the 13 high-risk strains (meaning a high chance of being 'oncogenic' – or encouraging cancer) of HPV develop cancer. It develops, for example, in less than 1 per cent of young women infected with high-risk HPV. In contrast, over 99 per cent of women who actually have cancer are infected with high-risk HPV (50 per cent with type 16 and 30% with types 18, 31 or 45) and low–risk HPV is rarely found in women with cancer.

The Pill

Studies over 30 years suggest that taking the combined Pill for more than five years almost doubles the risk of cervix cancer but only in certain women with other risk factors. What's nearly always necessary is a sexually transmitted infection of the cervix with human papillomaviruses (HPV), plus one or more other factors – such as smoking, starting sex young, having multiple sexual partners or taking the Pill.

Other risk factors

These include smoking; having pre-cancerous cells on the cervix; having poor immunity and taking the Pill for more than five years (see below). Chlamydia, herpesvirus infection, Epstein-Barr virus infection, and HIV infection may also encourage cervix cancer. There's also a suggestion that an uncircumcised sexual partner who doesn't keep his penis clean may increase your risk, owing to your cervix cells being sensitive to the secretions under his foreskin.

what to do yourself

To help *prevent* any cancer, lead a healthy lifestyle, minimise controllable risk factors, have any recommended screening; and report unexplained symptoms early.

To help *treat* cancer, lead a healthy lifestyle and minimise controllable risk factors, as some of these may influence cancer growth.

Screening – Routine screening with a cervical smear is advisable at certain ages since it identifies abnormal cells that might develop into cancer, so need a biopsy and either observation or treatment. Unfortunately, though, smears are not completely reliable; indeed, one in two women who get cervix cancer have had regular smears.

Most women with an abnormal smear certainly don't necessarily have cancer, however, their risk is raised. Depending on the findings and your history, you may need a repeat smear straight away, or more frequent repeat smears, until your smear is normal again. You may also need a colposcopy and, if necessary, a biopsy of your cervix.

It's likely that having an HPV test along with a routine smear will be introduced in developed countries in the next few years. One day, hopefully, there will be an HPV vaccine to help prevent infection.

A screening test called 'liquid-based cytology', in which cervix cells are put into a liquid before being sent to the lab, is being investigated as an alternative to a smear, as it seems to be around 80 per cent more reliable. Other screening developments being investigated include the use of a device that identifies abnormal cells by measuring how they react to light and pulses of electricity.

Safer sex – Ideally, only ever have sex with one faithful partner who is free from HPV infection. Otherwise, always use a condom unless you are sure that your partner is free from HPV infection and is faithful to you. Also, encourage your partner to keep his penis clean.

Consider an HPV test if on the Pill – If you take the Pill, and suspect that you may have HPV infection (perhaps because you've had many sexual partners and haven't always used a condom) consider asking your doctor for an HPV test. The combination of the Pill and HPV encourages cervix cancer, so if you're HPV-positive, it may be better to use another form of contraception.

No smoking – Smoking increases the risk of cervix cancer, so it's best to avoid it altogether – especially if you have a positive HPV test. It's possible, but unproven, that passive smoking increases the risk too.

Take general anti-cancer measures – See Gynae cancers, page 84.

Dietary changes – In addition to those mentioned in the general anti-cancer measures, eat plenty of foods rich in beta-carotene, vitamin C and folic acid, as these are particularly associated with healthy cervix cells.

Hydrotherapy – Have a daily contrast sitz bath (see page 275) to stimulate the circulation to your cervix and encourage healing.

Tests and investigations

If abnormal cells are detected in a routine smear, then – depending on the degree of the changes – you'll either need a repeat smear (immediately or sooner than you would otherwise have had your next one) or you'll need a colposcopy and biopsies to confirm the degree of abnormality in your cervix. If the doctor dabs dilute acetic acid (vinegar) on your cervix, any abnormal cells will turn whiter than usual.

need to see a doctor?

Yes, for regular screening with cervical smears. Yes if you suspect HPV infection and are on the Pill. And yes, if you have abnormal vaginal bleeding or some other reason to suspect cancer. The earlier you start medical treatment for this cancer, the more successful treatment is likely to be.

If a repeat smear reveals cells with mildly abnormal changes (mild dyskaryosis) a biopsy of the covering (epithelial) cells of the cervix generally shows cell changes called CIN 1 (cervical intraepithelial neoplasia, grade 1) – changes in the superficial third of the covering. If a smear reveals moderately abnormal cells (moderate dyskaryosis) a biopsy generally shows CIN 2-cell changes in the upper two-thirds. If a smear reveals severely abnormal cells (severe dyskaryosis) a biopsy generally shows CIN 3-cell changes throughout the whole thickness.

If your smear shows mild or abnormal cell changes your doctor may advise an HPV test. If this is negative you may not need such frequent repeat smears as you would if it were positive. If it's positive there's a chance the infection will clear spontaneously so, if it's safe to do so, your doctor may recommend postponing treatment of abnormal cells and repeating your HPV test in, perhaps, six months or so.

Medical treatment

HPV infection – Researchers are investigating the effectiveness of treating the cervix with a cream containing imiquimod, which alters the local immune response.

Abnormal cells – Cervix cells that are persistently mildly abnormal, or that are moderately or severely abnormal, are treated during colposcopy. The cervix is numbed with local anaesthetic. Then, depending on the extent and severity of the abnormality and on any previous treatment, the cervix is treated in one of two ways:

● The abnormal cells are 'ablated', which means destroyed, usually under local anaesthetic. This is done by cauterising them with silver nitrate; burning them with an electrically heated wire (loop diathermy) or a laser beam; or treating them with 'cold coagulation' (which actually uses heat to destroy the abnormal cells) or cryosurgery (which uses liquid nitrogen to freeze abnormal cells).

● If the doctor can't see all of the abnormal area because it extends into the cervical canal, he or she does a 'cone biopsy' under general anaesthetic. This is not a biopsy as such but the cutting out of a cone-shaped chunk of cervix tissue from around the lower two-thirds of the cervical canal, to be sure that all the abnormal cells are removed. Afterwards you may experience some pain and bleeding and a discharge. You should avoid heavy lifting and over-exertion for two or three weeks. Avoid penetrative sex for at least six weeks.

Cancer – Treatment depends on a cancer's stage and the earlier a cancer is detected the more successful this is likely to be. Overall, around 74 per cent of women treated for cervix cancer in Australia and the US are alive after five years (and the figures are even better in Iceland, though not as good in other European countries, including the UK). However, US figures, for example, show that 80-95 per cent of women with stage-1 cancer (meaning cancer confined to the cervix) survive longer than five years. In contrast, only 20 per cent of women with stage-4 cancer (meaning their cancer has spread beyond their pelvic cavity or into their bladder or rectum) survive that long.

Treatment is with some combination of hysterectomy, radiotherapy, anti-cancer drugs (chemotherapy), and other medication.

Researchers are investigating laser destruction of cancer cells that have been sensitised with a light-absorbing pigment. Other promising new research, albeit at an extremely early stage, involves the idea of using gene therapy to destroy cancer cells.

A new operation involves removing only the cervix and leaving the rest of the womb. Not only is this just as successful as removing the whole womb, in terms of getting rid of early cervix cancer that hasn't yet spread outside the cervix, but it's unlikely to prevent a woman from having a baby later.

your action plan

✔ **Vital**

- Medical observation or treatment
- Safer sex
- No smoking
- General anti-cancer measures (page 84)

- Dietary changes
- Minimise controllable risk factors

(✔) **Optional**

- Hydrotherapy

womb cancer

Each year in the UK, the USA and other westernised countries, up to one woman in 5,000 discovers that she has this cancer (also called endometrial or uterine cancer). Womb cancer is very rare in women under 40 and most common over 60. Women who take the combined contraceptive Pill are less likely to get it, as are women who are mothers.

You may have heavy periods or bleeding between periods; if you've stopped having periods, the most likely symptom is post-menopausal bleeding. Other possibilities include pain low in your abdomen and during sex and a vaginal discharge. Advanced cancer can cause loss of appetite and weight, tiredness, weakness, nausea, vomiting, constipation, frequent urination and pain in the back or legs.

Factors that can encourage womb cancer include anything associated with an oestrogen-dominant hormone imbalance and large numbers of menstrual cycles during a woman's reproductive life. So cancer is more likely if you are overweight or have irregular periods or an abnormally thick womb lining (which shows up as heavy periods, bleeding between periods, or post-menopausal bleeding). It's also more likely if you've had no children, are infertile from ovarian failure, haven't breastfed, have a late menopause or take badly prescribed HRT (containing only oestrogen), especially if you take it for a long time.

Another possible risk factor is tamoxifen, taken to help prevent or treat oestrogen-dependent breast cancer. For while tamoxifen can protect the breasts from a woman's own, stronger oestrogen, its own oestrogenic effects – although mild – are enough to stimulate the womb lining. The risk to women on tamoxifen doubles if they take it for two to five years and multiplies sevenfold if they're on it longer. It's essential to tell your doctor if you have any abnormal bleeding when on tamoxifen.

A close family history of bowel, breast, ovary or womb cancer also raises your risk of womb cancer, as does having polycystic ovary syndrome, high blood pressure, or diabetes. Womb cancer in women under 35 is usually due to a failure to ovulate because of polycystic ovary syndrome or an oestrogen-producing tumour.

Fortunately, womb cancer is usually discovered early, when treatment is highly likely to result in a cure.

what to do yourself

To help prevent cancer, lead a healthy lifestyle; minimise controllable risk factors; and report unexplained symptoms early.

To treat cancer, lead a healthy lifestyle, and minimise controllable risk factors – as some of these may influence cancer growth.

Take general anti-cancer measures – see 'Gynae cancers', page 84.

Discourage oestrogen dominance – (see page 89), with dietary changes, regular exercise, healthy-weight maintenance, and the avoidance of xeno-oestrogens.

Tests and investigations

An ultrasound scan may be advised and a Pipelle womb biopsy or a biopsy done through a hysteroscope, is done to detect womb cancer.

Until recently it hasn't been clear how best to screen for early womb cancer in women taking tamoxifen but new research shows that a regular womb biopsy for this purpose is unnecessary,

need to see a doctor?

There is no suitable screening test for the general population. However, if your risk is high because you have a family history of certain cancers, discuss with your doctor whether a regular ultrasound scan or womb-lining (endometrial) biopsy is advisable.

You must see a doctor if you have abnormal vaginal bleeding or any other worrying symptom.

since abnormal bleeding indicates womb cancer just as reliably.

Medical treatment

The usual treatment is a total hysterectomy (removal of the womb, cervix and fallopian tubes). Sometimes this is followed by radiotherapy. However, one trial shows that many women whose cancer hasn't yet spread beyond their womb don't need radiotherapy to boost their chance of survival. Radiotherapy alone may be wise for women with advanced cancer. Ongoing research aims to discover whether anti-cancer medication (chemotherapy) is helpful.

In the USA, around 85 per cent of women treated for womb cancer survive for at least five years (95 per cent if it is picked up very early); the figure in Australia is around 81 per cent, while in the UK, it is over 70 per cent.

your action plan

✔ **Vital**

• Medical treatment

• Take general anti-cancer measures (see page 84)

• Discourage oestrogen dominance (see page 89)

• Avoid controllable risk factors

vulva and vagina

Your vulva and vagina are lined with cells that are more delicate and produce more moisture than those in the skin. It's helpful to use a mirror to look at and get to know your vulva so that you can spot anything unusual (don't worry at all if it doesn't resemble the stylised drawings you have seen in health books). Feeling inside your vagina with your fingers – crouching if necessary – will help you to detect soreness or lumps.

lump in the vulva or vagina

In the vulva

One possibility is a sebaceous cyst, formed by a blockage of one of the skin-oil (sebum) producing glands in the hairy outer surface of one of the outer lips. Others include a boil, varicose veins, genital warts, inflamed Bartholin's gland and cancer.

The Bartholin's glands produce a slippery fluid when you're sexually aroused and there's one each side of the vagina's opening. Normally you can't feel them, but if one becomes inflamed, you'll have a hot, red, swelling that's so painful it might prevent you from sitting. The inflammation usually results from infection and might make you feel unwell and feverish. The inflammation will probably get better by itself but there's a chance it may form an abscess requiring urgent treatment or develop into a fluid-filled cyst that keeps becoming inflamed.

In the vagina

Possibilities include a cervix or womb polyp on a stalk, a fibroid on a stalk, a prolapse and a cancer – though this is rare.

what to do yourself

For an inflamed Bartholin's gland

Act early to help prevent an abscess from forming, as this can be difficult to treat.

Dietary changes – Eat a healthy diet for beta-carotene, vitamins C and E, selenium, zinc, plant pigments, and other nutrients that help to counteract infection. Also, eat more foods rich in omega-3 fatty acids and less of those rich in omega-6s, although you should reduce your overall intake of fat, especially the saturated type, to help reduce inflammation.

No smoking – Smoking reduces immunity so stop or, at least, cut right down and try to avoid passive smoking.

Exercise – Take half an hour's daily 'whole-body' exercise, such as brisk walking, to aid healing by boosting your pelvic circulation.

Massage – Twice a day, massage the inflamed gland with your fingertips, pinching it from underneath and gently but firmly moving your fingertips up to meet on top. Repeat several times to help release any blockage in the gland's duct. Don't do this massage if the gland is very painful though.

symptom sorter

Gynae or gynae-related causes of lump in vulva

- ••• **Most likely** – sebaceous cyst, boil, inflamed Bartholin's gland
- •• **Less likely** – genital warts
- • **Possible** – varicose veins, vulva cancer

Gynae or gynae-related causes of lump in vagina

- ••• **Most likely** – prolapse
- •• **Less likely** – womb or cervix polyp, fibroid (on a stalk)
- • **Possible** – forgotten tampon or diaphragm, stools in rectum felt through the vagina's wall, vagina cancer

Fresh air – Go without knickers whenever you can until the area heals, as fresh air encourages healing.

Hydrotherapy and aromatherapy – Soak for half an hour each day in a warm bath containing two drops each of tea tree and juniper oils, as these are antiseptic. Also, have a daily contrast sitz bath (see page 275) to boost your pelvic circulation and aid healing.

Herbal remedies – Apply arnica cream twice a day to help prevent infection and aid healing.

Cold – If a very tense abscess develops apply an ice pack for a minute or two to help relieve pain

Painkillers – If you have a tense abscess take over-the-counter painkillers if necessary.

Food supplements – Consider taking a supplement containing beta-carotene, vitamins C and E, selenium and zinc to help counteract infection and fish oil for any inflammation. Plant pigments such as lycopene and flavonoids may help too, because of their antioxidant action.

Tests and investigations

Your doctor may recommend treatment straight away and send a swab from the lump to a laboratory to be tested for the type of infecting micro-organisms and the most suitable antibiotics. If there's any possibility of cancer, a gynaecologist can take a biopsy (sample) for the laboratory to examine.

need to see a doctor?

Yes, if you don't know what the lump is, if home treatments do not start working within a week, if the pain is severe, you feel generally unwell or if the lump grows. Very occasionally cancer masquerades as a swollen Bartholin's gland.

Medical treatment

For an inflamed Bartholin's gland you can start an antibiotic at once and change to another if the laboratory findings suggest this is better. For an abscess, you may need a small operation to allow the pus to drain. For an abscess which keeps recurring, or a cyst which repeatedly becomes inflamed, an operation called marsupialisation, done under local or general anaesthetic, can prevent further problems by permanently opening the gland.

your action plan

For an inflamed Bartholin's gland

✔ **Vital**

• Dietary changes

• No smoking

• Exercise

✔ **Could be vital**

• Medical assessment and treatment

• Massage

• Fresh air

• Hydrotherapy and aromatherapy

• Herbal remedies

(✔) **Optional**

• Cold

• Painkillers

• Food supplements

For other problems

✔ **Could be vital**

• Medical assessment

• Appropriate home and medical
  treatments

sore, itchy vulva and sore vagina

perhaps with a vaginal discharge

An inflamed vulva is known as 'vulvitis', and an inflamed vagina 'vaginitis'. If both vulva and vagina are affected, it's 'vulvo-vaginitis'.

In premenopausal women the most common causes of an abnormal vaginal discharge and inflammation are bacterial vaginosis and candida infection of the vagina and vulva. Sexually transmitted or other infections can cause inflammation and a discharge but itching is less likely to occur. A foreign body in the vagina, such as a forgotten tampon or diaphragm, or, in young children, any small object poked in out of curiosity, can become infected, leading to inflammation and a smelly discharge. Very occasionally, an inflamed vagina and vaginal discharge signify a cervical 'erosion', or cervix cancer.

symptom sorter

Gynae or gynae-related causes of sore and, perhaps, itchy vulva

● ● ● **Most likely** – vigorous sex with poor lubrication, candida infection, diabetes

● ● **Less likely** – sensitivity to a toiletry or washing power, psoriasis, eczema, thyroid disorder, genital-wart virus infection, herpes infection, lichen sclerosis

● **Possible** – leukoplakia, anaemia, aphthous ulcers, threadworms, scabies, pubic lice, Behçet's disease, injury, vulva cancer, cancer elsewhere

Gynae or gynae-related causes of sore vagina

● ● ● **Most likely** – vigorous sex with poor lubrication, bacterial vaginosis, candida infection, sexually transmitted infection

● ● **Less likely** – allergy to latex in condom or sex toy or to spermicide; episiotomy; foreign body; atrophic vulvo-vaginitis

● **Possible** – cervix or vagina cancer

Gynae or gynae-related causes of vaginal discharge

● ● ● **Most likely** – can be normal in second half of cycle, menstrual loss, bacterial vaginosis, candida infection, sexually transmitted infection.

● ● **Less likely** – oestrogen dominance, cervical 'erosion', inflamed cervix, foreign body.

● **Possible** – pelvic inflammatory disease, womb or cervix polyp, cervix cancer.

Several skin conditions, including psoriasis and eczema, can make the vulva itchy, as can infestation with scabies mites or pubic lice ('crabs') and certain general conditions such as diabetes, iron-deficiency anaemia, thyroid disorders and lymphoma and other cancers. A condition called leukoplakia creates itchy white patches of thickened, cracked skin in the vulva; these are occasionally pre-cancerous and can spread to involve the back passage. Itching may also be associated with normal-looking pre-cancerous tissue that is likely to be infected with wart viruses (see HPV, page 204). With 'lichen sclerosis', in which elastin in the skin's elastic fibres is replaced with more rigid collagen, areas of the vulva appear white, flat and shiny and feel intensely itchy. This is most likely to occur in postmenopausal women, in whom it occasionally develops into cancer and in pre-adolescent girls, in whom there's a 50:50 chance that it will disappear at puberty. Another cause of itchy inflammation is sensitivity to a toiletry product such as perfumed talcum powder or deodorant or to traces of washing powder in knickers. In a young girl threadworms can irritate the vulva and around the anus. Soreness of the vulva may be due to painful 'aphthous' ulcers (like common mouth ulcers). Another possibility is Behçet's disease, which can make the vulva intensely and embarrassingly itchy and also cause mouth ulcers, arthritis and pain in the eyes; it's associated with an overactive immune system and, while its cause is unknown, viral infection is under suspicion.

Inflammation can also result from an injury to the vulva or vagina (such as from an uncomfortable bicycle saddle, over-enthusiastic sex, or sexual abuse.

After the menopause the most common cause of soreness is atrophic vulvo-vaginitis, associated with a low level of oestrogen (see urethral syndrome, under 'Dry vagina and vulva', page 173). This thins and dries the surface of the vulva and vagina encouraging inflammation and, perhaps, a discharge but it doesn't make you itch.

what to do yourself

Avoid toiletries on your vulva – Any product might be irritating, especially if perfumed. If you suspect toiletries, avoid using them for three weeks to see if your symptoms settle.

Use appropriate home remedies – once you know the cause.

Adjust laundering – Wash knickers and trousers at as high a temperature as possible and wear cotton knickers you can launder in very hot water. If you suspect a 'biological' washing powder (one with enzymes) or a fabric conditioner to be the cause, try a 'non-biological' powder and omit conditioner.

Use aqueous cream to clean your vulva, not soap – which may encourage itching.

Avoid sex – if this is painful, or you suspect a sexually transmitted infection.

Lose excess weight – as this makes itching worse.

Tests and investigations

Your doctor will look at your vulva and take swabs from your vulva, vagina or cervix, if necessary, so the laboratory can check the nature of the infection and the antibiotics that will help. It's wise to have a cervical smear and a diabetes test. If your doctor thinks cancer is a possibility, he or she will refer you to a gynaecologist for colposcopy. If you have leukoplakia, your gynaecologist will do a biopsy and regular checks.

need to see a doctor?

Yes, if home treatment doesn't work, if you don't know what's wrong, if you suspect a sexually transmitted infection or if your symptoms are severe or continue for more than a week. If you have lichen sclerosis, see your doctor for regular cancer checks.

Medical treatment

This depends on the cause. A mild steroid cream may help lichen sclerosis but should be used sparingly as steroids can thin the skin and be absorbed into the body.

your action plan

✔ **Vital**
• Avoid toiletries on your vulva

✔ **Could be vital**
• Medical assessment
• Appropriate home and medical treatments
• Adjusting laundering

• Using aqueous cream
• Avoiding sex
• Losing excess weight

dry vagina and vulva

Normally the vulva and vagina keep themselves moist. Moisture production rises around ovulation and decreases for a few days before and after a period. It rises during sexual arousal, may fall for some months after childbirth and often lessens a year or two after the menopause.

Dryness can lead to soreness, discomfort during sex and urgent and frequent urination; it can also make you more vulnerable to injury and infection. Certain formulations of the Pill can make the vagina and vulva less moist. Three other causes are Sjögren's (pronounced 'show-grens') syndrome; a high prolactin level (see 'Nipple itching and/or discharge, page 70) and atrophic vulvo-vaginitis.

Sjögren's – Moisture-producing glands throughout the body become inflamed, leading to widespread dryness – especially in the vagina, eyes, nose and mouth. Other possible problems include fatigue and Raynaud's phenomenon (painful blue fingers in sudden cold weather). There's a raised risk of a connective tissue disorder (such as rheumatoid arthritis, lupus, or inflamed blood vessels – vasculitis), disorders of the nerves, liver, pancreas, kidneys or bones and a lymphoma (lymph-tissue cancer).

Sjögren's tends to come and go and is an autoimmune condition. Possible triggers include physical or mental stresses and genetic factors and there's an increased risk of having raised levels of gluten antibodies, suggesting that gluten sensitivity might be a trigger. Nine out of 10 people with Sjögren's are women, most are over 40 and it affects up to 3 per cent of 50-70-year-olds.

Atrophic vulvo-vaginitis – This means that the lining of the vagina and vulva are thin and dry, which encourages soreness and inflammation; it's most common after the menopause and results from a low oestrogen level. Some women with atrophic vulvo-vaginitis also have thinning of the lining of the urethra, causing cystitis-like symptoms known as the **urethral syndrome**, with urgent, frequent, painful urination but no urine infection.

what to do yourself

Pinpoint and prevent Sjögren's triggers – if possible.

Keep well hydrated – Avoid salty or salted foods, alcohol and coffee – and drink plenty of water and water-based fluids.

Dietary changes – Eat a healthy, varied diet to encourage good moisture production and immunity (especially if you have Sjögren's) and good oestrogen production for your age (especially if you have atrophic vulvo-vaginitis). Include foods rich in plant oestrogens. Also, have plenty of foods rich in beta-carotene and vitamins B6, C and E and eat more food rich in omega-3 fatty acids and less rich in omega-6s to reduce any inflammation.

symptom sorter

Gynae or gynae-related causes of dry vagina and vulva

● ● ● **Most likely** – oestrogen deficient hormone imbalance (for example, after the menopause and on certain formulations of Pill)

● **Possible** – Sjögren's syndrome

Sexual arousal and lubrication – During sex, take whatever time you need to become aroused. The more often you become aroused, the more moisture you'll make, and regular orgasms help too. If necessary, lubricate with saliva, almond oil, or a commercial vaginal lubricant (such as K-Y jelly).

Pelvic floor exercises – Each day, do pelvic floor exercises to boost the circulation to your vagina and vulva (see page 265).

Healthy weight maintenance – Avoid becoming too thin, especially if you have atrophic vulvo-vaginitis, as a low body weight reduces the body's oestrogen level.

Exercise – Take half-an-hour's daily exercise to boost the circulation to your vulva, vagina, and hormone-producing glands. However, avoid over-exercising, especially if you have atrophic vulvo-vaginitis, as this reduces the body's oestrogen level.

Light and dark – Each day, you should be exposed to at least 15 minutes of bright outdoor daylight to encourage healthy hormone balance. Also, make sure, particularly if you have Sjögren's, that you get enough sleep in a dark room, as this enables the pineal to produce melatonin, which boosts immunity and helps prevent soreness due to infection.

No smoking – particularly if you have atrophic vulvo-vaginitis, as smoking encourages the production of less active oestrogens (such as oestrone).

Herbal remedies – If you have atrophic vulvo-vaginitis, drink a cup of fennel or sage tea each day. Alternatively, try black cohosh, as studies show its plant oestrogens are as effective as the oestrogen in HRT, or try *Vitex agnus castus*. Other remedies rich in plant oestrogens include red clover and a concentrate made from soy beans or tofu (from health stores and some pharmacies).

Alternatively, try a vaginal gel containing a soy extract (see the Helplist, page 315). One study of women over 50 found this improved the moisture content of vagina lining cells by 36 per cent and their elasticity by nearly 40 per cent and doubled moisture production.

Food supplements – Some women with atrophic vulvo-vaginitis find vitamins B6, C and E helpful.

Hydrotherapy – Once or twice a week, have a contrast sitz bath (see page 275) to boost the circulation in your vulva and vagina.

Aromatherapy – If you have atrophic vulvo-vaginitis add two drops each of geranium and sweet fennel oils to your bath water and soak for half an hour. These oils are believed to stimulate the production of female sex hormones.

Tests and investigations

Your doctor may take swabs to check there's no infection and, if necessary, measure the vagina's acidity, as an unusually low level (pH over 4.5) is a feature of atrophic vulvo-vaginitis. Blood tests for autoantibodies can help to diagnose Sjögren's.

need to see a doctor?
Yes, if home remedies aren't enough to overcome problems due to dryness.

Medical treatment

There's no cure for Sjögren's but some combination of non-steroidal anti-inflammatory drugs, steroids and certain other drugs will relieve severe symptoms.

If you are on the Pill, discuss taking a more oestrogenic formulation or using different contraception.

For atrophic vulvo-vaginitis, your doctor may suggest oestrogen-containing vaginal cream or pessaries (vaginal tablets) or an oestrogen-containing ring replaced in your vagina every three months. The response to this low-potency, 'topical' oestrogen is usually dramatic and unlikely to cause any worrying thickening of the womb lining. However, if you use it for more than three months, discuss whether you need to take a progestogen to reduce your risk of womb cancer. Reassuringly, although some oestrogen is absorbed into the bloodstream from the vulva and vagina, Swedish and American researchers recently showed this doesn't increase the risk of womb cancer. Surprisingly, perhaps, taking HRT (hormone replacement therapy) tablets or patches does not improve the symptoms.

If you have urethral syndrome, other troublesome menopausal signs or a raised risk of osteoporosis, your doctor may prescribe HRT instead of topical oestrogen. If so, unless you've had a hysterectomy, your HRT must contain a progestogen, as well as oestrogen, to counteract the raised risk of womb cancer from oestrogen alone.

your action plan

✔ Vital

- Pinpoint Sjögren's triggers
- Keep well hydrated
- Dietary changes
- Sex – arousal and lubrication
- Pelvic floor exercises
- Healthy weight maintenance
- Exercise
- Exposure to light and darkness

✔ Could be vital

- Medical treatment
- No smoking
- Herbal remedies

(✔) Optional

- Food supplements
- Hydrotherapy
- Aromatherapy

bacterial vaginosis

This common condition is caused by an overgrowth of organisms normally present in the vagina. It usually means *Gardnerella vaginalis* bacteria have ousted the protective lactobacilli. Bacterial vaginosis occurs almost exclusively in sexually active women but is not a sexually transmitted infection. Its only symptom is a greyish-white, sticky vaginal discharge with a fishy smell. Bacterial vaginosis is more likely to be responsible for a vaginal discharge than is candida infection so, if you think you have candida and are treating yourself with home and over-the-counter remedies, see your doctor if your symptoms don't improve.

Bacterial vaginosis is sometimes triggered by the presence of a coil and other causes include antibiotics, vaginal deodorants and douching. It's likely to go spontaneously in time but at worst it can encourage pelvic inflammatory disease and, in pregnancy, miscarriage or pre-term birth.

what to do yourself

General good health – Encourage healing with a healthy diet, regular exercise, no smoking, daily exposure to bright outside light, enough sleep, and effective stress management. Have regular cervical smears, as bacterial vaginosis can encourage abnormal cervix cells.

Avoid vaginal douching – This upsets the normal balance of micro-organisms and is not necessary.

Tests and investigations

Your doctor may look at a sample of your vaginal discharge under a microscope to detect characteristic 'clue cells'. A pH (acidity level) test may aid diagnosis, as bacterial vaginosis usually makes the vagina less acidic than normal. The

need to see a doctor?

Yes, if you have an abnormal and ongoing vaginal discharge.

'whiff' test, in which the doctor puts two drops of potassium hydroxide on a drop of the discharge, can be useful; a fishy smell suggests bacterial vaginosis. Your doctor will send swabs from your vagina to a laboratory to check the nature of the infection, to determine which antibiotics will be effective.

Medical treatment

Non-pregnant women can use a vaginal gel containing metronidazole, or an antibacterial vaginal cream containing clindamycin.

Pregnant women need tablets of an antibiotic called metronidazole.

your action plan

✔ **Vital**
- Medical treatment
- Avoid vaginal douching

✔ **Could be vital**
- General good health measures

candida infection

Infection of the vagina with the yeast-like fungus *Candida albicans* causes intense itching, inflammation, soreness, and a creamy-white, curd-like discharge. It usually involves the vulva too. Sometimes it is called thrush, and some women have repeated attacks.

Candida is a normal inhabitant of the vulva, vagina and bowel but if it multiplies too much it causes infection. It can also infect the inside of the mouth (especially in a breastfeeding baby or a very unwell person), a breastfeeding woman's nipples and the sides of the nails. A bowel infection can damage the bowel lining, allowing particles of undigested food to enter the lymph system and blood and so encouraging food sensitivity. Very occasionally, in very ill – usually hospitalised – people, candida actually enters the blood, causing generalised infection (invasive candidiasis). This can damage the kidneys, liver and other organs, and kills up to two in five affected people.

Infection is most common in sexually active women and is sometimes spread during sex. It can be triggered by antibiotics, stress, poor immunity, steroid drugs, and changing hormone levels (in pregnancy, around the menopause and when on the Pill or HRT). Unrecognised or poorly controlled diabetes encourages infection because candida thrives on a high sugar level.

what to do yourself

Wear cotton knickers, avoid tight trousers – This helps by increasing the airflow around the vulva and reducing the high humidity that candida likes.

Dietary changes – Boost immunity with foods rich in beta-carotene, vitamins C and E, selenium, zinc and flavonoids. Eat several raw garlic cloves each day, for example, in a salad dressing, or take garlic capsules, to help control infection. Each day, drink a liquidised grapefruit, complete with peel, pith and pips, for its natural antifungal agents, or take grapefruit-seed extract tablets (from health stores).

Drink less alcohol and cut down on foods containing sugar or white flour, which encourage candida.

Use anti-fungal medication – from the pharmacist. This could be antifungal clotrimazole pessaries and cream, or one capsule of an antifungal drug called fluconazole (though not if you're pregnant, under 16, or over 60). Note that antifungal creams and pessaries can damage condoms and diaphragms.

Avoid toiletries for your vulva and vagina – These may further irritate inflamed areas.

Avoid panty liners between periods – Avoid liners between periods since their plastic backing increases heat and humidity, which encourages candida.

Launder carefully – Wash bed linen, towels and clothes in very hot water and rinse well. Don't share towels, or flannels.

Avoid perfumed soap – Wash your vulva using unperfumed soap or clean yourself with aqueous cream (from a pharmacy) to avoid further irritation.

Garlic and lactobacillus pessaries – Consider trying Yeastguard (see the Helplist, page 315) pessaries (vaginal tablets), which contain an odourless garlic extract, allicin, along with *Lactobacillus acidophilus* bacteria. Laboratory tests show allicin rapidly kills candida and the (unproven) idea is that the lactobacilli will prevent further candida overgrowth by rebalancing the normal balance of micro-organisms in the vagina.

Yoghurt – For many years natural therapists and some doctors recommended inserting a tampon soaked in live yoghurt twice a day in the hope that the yoghurt's lactobacilli would help to restore a natural balance of micro-organisms in the vagina. They also suggested eating live yoghurt each day to restore a normal balance of micro-organisms in the gut, in case the vagina was repeatedly being infected by candida from an overgrowth in the gut travelling from the anus into the vulva and vagina. These were interesting theories but, unfortunately, relatively recent studies have shown that neither inserting yoghurt-soaked tampons nor eating yoghurt helps to cure vaginal thrush.

Food supplements – Consider taking vitamins A, C, E, zinc, to boost immunity and dampen inflammation. Grapefruit seed extract may help too as it has antifungal activity.

Hydrotherapy and aromatherapy – On alternate days add six drops of tea tree oil, or a handful of salt plus a cup of unpasteurised apple cider vinegar (from a health store), to your bath water and soak in it for half an hour.

Herbal remedies – Beth root or echinacea may help. Try soothing itching with goldenseal tea.

(Note the advice on page 277 when using herbal remedies.)

Tests and investigations

A doctor can see the yeast-like organisms by putting a drop of vaginal fluid under the microscope. There are specific laboratory tests for candida but these take time and detect fewer than one in two cases, so many doctors prefer to make an educated guess and begin treatment straight away. A test of the vagina's acidity level (pH) helps to distinguish candida infection from bacterial vaginosis – if you have bacterial vaginosis your vagina has a relatively high pH (as it's much less acidic than normal). Your doctor may do a urine-sugar test for diabetes.

need to see a doctor?

Yes, if your symptoms continue for more than a week in spite of home treatment, or keep recurring. Your partner may need treatment too.

Medical treatment

Your doctor may recommend oral or vaginal clotrimazole, oral fluconazole, or vaginal nystatin. If these do not help within a week or so, it is likely that something else is causing your symptoms. Indeed, one in three women with typical candida symptoms turns out not to have candida. Your partner may need treatment too, although proof that this would help to clear up your infection, or prevent re-infection, is lacking.

your action plan

✔ **Vital**

- Wear cotton knickers and avoid tight trousers
- Dietary changes
- Use antifungal medication
- Avoid toiletries for your vulva and vagina
- Avoid panty liners between periods
- Launder carefully
- Avoid perfumed soap
- Reduce controllable risk factors

✔ **Could be vital**

- Medical treatment

(✔) **Optional**

- Garlic and lactobacillus pessaries
- Food supplements
- Hydrotherapy and aromatherapy
- Herbal remedies

vulva cancer

This is rare and occurs mostly in elderly women. It usually starts with an itchy, thickened, white, red or otherwise discoloured patch of pre-cancerous cells. There may also be soreness, burning pain on passing urine (if the surface is sore), a discharge, bleeding or a growth although, sometimes, pre-cancerous cells are symptom-free. One in five women with pre-cancerous cells develops cancer within 10 years. Without effective treatment vulva cancer can destroy underlying tissues and may eventually cause more widespread damage, or kill.

Risk factors include smoking, ageing and infection with human papillomaviruses (HPV). Indeed, between a third and a half of all women with vulva cancer have HPV infection – usually with high-risk types of virus (see page 204). Other risk factors include certain skin problems, including lichen sclerosis and leukoplakia (see page 171) and, perhaps, poor hygiene.

A few vulva cancers are malignant melanomas which in other areas would be attributed to too much sun but, since the vulva doesn't see much sun, other factors must encourage them.

what to do yourself

To help prevent this cancer lead a healthy lifestyle, minimise controllable risk factors and report unexplained symptoms early. Sexually active women should practise 'safer sex'.

There is no routine screening for vulva cancer but the doctor will look at your vulva when you have your routine cervical smear and you can look at your vulva in a mirror if you suspect a problem (see page 167).

To help *treat* vulva cancer, again lead a healthy lifestyle and minimise controllable risk factors – as some of these may influence cancer growth.

Take general anti-cancer measures – See Gynae cancers, page 84.

Non-smoking – as smoking encourages vulva cancer.

need to see a doctor?

Yes, without delay, if any of the above symptoms is unexplained.

Tests and investigations

Your doctor will examine your vulva and take a biopsy if necessary. Cancer cells infected with HPV whiten for longer, and more deeply, than do normal ones when dabbed with dilute acetic acid (vinegar). If high-risk types of HPV are present your doctor will see you for an annual check and cervical smear. One woman in 10 with vulva cancer associated with HPV has another cancer elsewhere, most often on her cervix, so regular cervix and breast checks are particularly important.

Medical treatment

Pre-cancerous patches can be treated with 5-fluorouracil cream or simple surgery. A newer treatment is available involving taking a light-sensitising substance called a psoralen then having ultraviolet light shone on the patches. Another possibility is destruction of the cancer with laser light.

Treatment of all but the smallest actual cancers involves surgery and frequent follow-ups are essential as this cancer may recur.

your action plan

✔ **Vital**

- Medical treatments
- General anti-cancer measures (see page 84)
- Non-smoking
- Minimise controllable risk factors

pelvis

The pelvic cavity lies between the pelvic bones at either side of your body, the base of the spine at the back, and the pubic bone (beneath the pubic hair) in front. It contains the upper reproductive tract (womb and tubes) and the lower reproductive tract (vagina), as well as the vulva. Most health concerns involving the reproductive tract and vulva are discussed elsewhere, so we will concentrate here on pelvic pain and pelvic inflammatory disease.

pelvic pain

Pelvic pain is as common as migraine, asthma and back pain and more likely to occur as we get older. One UK report found that nearly 3 per cent of women over 60 have it each month, compared with nearly 2 per cent of 15-20 year-olds. It can be a real nuisance with one woman in three finding it persists for at least two years after seeing her doctor about it for the first time.

Many factors can cause pelvic pain. Irritable bowel syndrome and cystitis commonly accompany long-term pelvic pain and may also cause it. Period pains and pain during sex are also more likely in women with long-term pelvic pain. Women with chronic fatigue syndrome are more likely to have pelvic pain. Less common causes include pain associated with ovulation, endometriosis, pelvic inflammatory disease, bowel or bladder cancer, advanced cervix cancer or a prolapse. Another possibility is adhesions associated with pelvic inflammatory disease, endometriosis, or following surgery (adhesions are strands of tissue associated with inflammation that can stick organs together; sometimes they cause pain by 'lassoing' an ovary – 'trapped ovary syndrome'). Pelvic congestion – resulting from a sluggish flow of blood and lymph overfilling veins and lymph vessels – causes an aching pain that is worse on standing or lifting, during sex, before a period and with a heavy period. It has been suggested that stress can encourage pelvic congestion by preventing the ovaries and pelvic blood vessels from working properly. Recent pelvic surgery or cervix treatments can cause pelvic pain and ovary cysts are a rare cause. Sometimes low abdominal pain is hard to distinguish from pelvic pain.

what to do yourself

Treat the cause, such as irritable bowel syndrome or cystitis (see page 223) if known.

Pelvic-floor exercises (see page 265), and pelvic-tilt exercises – These boost your pelvic circulation and help to prevent pain. You do pelvic-tilt exercises by kneeling on your hands and knees and rapidly rocking your lower back up and down for several minutes. Both exercises are especially useful for pelvic congestion.

Massage and aromatherapy – Gently massaging your tummy, lubricating with three or four drops of lavender oil in two teaspoons of sweet almond (or other carrier) oil, may help you to manage pain by easing physical and mental tension.

Mind techniques – Help yourself cope with the pain by finding effective ways of managing stress and distracting your mind.

Exercise – Take half an hour's daily whole-body exercise to boost your circulation and wellbeing and, perhaps, reduce pain, especially from pelvic congestion. This is particularly important if your lifestyle is largely sedentary.

Hydrotherapy – Each day have a contrast sitz bath (see page 275). This may be especially helpful for pelvic congestion.

Painkillers – Take over-the-counter remedies if necessary.

Tests and investigations

Your doctor will examine you, and may do blood, urine and pregnancy tests and an ultrasound scan. You may need a colposcopy, laparoscopy or venogram (an investigation to show how well your pelvic veins function). However, in one in two women investigated for long-term pelvic pain, no cause is found.

need to see a doctor?

Yes, if unexplained pain persists for more than a week or so, if it is severe or increasing or if you have other worrying symptoms. Report any unexplained weight loss, persistent diarrhoea or constipation, blood or mucus in your stools or a lump in your tummy. Ensure that you have regular smears.

symptom sorter

Gynae or gynae-related causes of pelvic pain

●●● **Most likely** – period pain, 'cystitis', irritable bowel syndrome, sexually transmitted infection, stress, inflamed cervix, womb or cervix polyp

●● **Less likely** – ovulation, endometriosis, pelvic inflammatory disease, bowel or bladder cancer, advanced cervix cancer, prolapse, pelvic congestion, adhesions

● **Possible** – ovary cyst, recent surgery or cervix treatment

Gynae or gynae-related caused of low abdominal pain – which is easily mistaken for pelvic pain

●●● **Most likely** – overweight (encouraging indigestion), irritable bowel

●● **Less likely** – endometriosis

● **Possible** – ovary cyst, fibroid (twisted), ovary or womb cancer

Medical treatment

This depends on the cause, and includes suggestions for managing the pain. Some doctors treat long-term pelvic congestion with progestogen to prevent ovulation, or with gonadotrophin-releasing hormone (gonadorelin) analogues – which eventually reduce the release of a woman's own ovary-stimulating hormones and so inhibit oestrogen production. This causes a reversible menopause whose symptoms can be treated with 'add-back' HRT. A new alternative, for some women is keyhole surgery to cut the nerves that carry pain messages from the womb, and a trial of this treatment is in progress.

your action plan

✔ **Could be vital**

- Mind techniques
- Pelvic-floor and pelvic-tilt exercises
- Massage
- Exercise
- Rest
- Hydrotherapy
- Painkillers
- Appropriate home and medical treatment

pelvic inflammatory disease

This is an infection of the womb, and/or fallopian tubes, and/or ovaries that may spread through the tubes, into the 'space' in the pelvis around the womb, bladder and large bowel. The infection causes inflammation. Pelvic inflammatory disease (PID) is the most frequent severe gynae infection and is more common in young women, those with a new sexual partner, and those who don't use condoms. Having a coil fitted while you have a chlamydia or other sexually transmitted infection can also encourage PID. Occasionally infection of the womb (endometritis) and the fallopian tubes (salpingitis) happens alone, but if the womb is infected, the tubes are likely to be infected too, and vice versa.

The first attack is usually the worst, with pelvic pain (that may be severe), fever, and flu-like symptoms – such as shivering, headache and aching muscles. Your cervix may be tender during sex (especially with deep penetration) and medical examinations, and you may feel pain in your thighs, bottom and lower back that's worse before a period. Your period may be unusually heavy. There may be a slight but smelly vaginal discharge (or, if your PID results from gonorrhoea, a yellow or bloody discharge). You may also have cystitis, and pain in your back passage. The pain can mimic that of endometriosis (see page 120). Also, the symptoms of salpingitis in the right fallopian tube mimic those of appendicitis, and symptoms from infection in either tube can be difficult to distinguish from an ectopic pregnancy (one occurring in a tube). If you feel nauseous, or vomit, you may have peritonitis (inflammation of the membranes around your abdominal organs).

If PID persists, its symptoms tend to become vaguer, periods may become painful, and in one in three women periods are heavy and, perhaps, frequent or irregular. Inflamed fallopian tubes can become kinked, blocked and scarred, impeding the passage of an egg. Without early and successful treatment, the tubes may become permanently blocked, or an abscess may develop in a tube (or, if the infection spreads into the pelvis, on an ovary). The result is a higher risk of ectopic pregnancy or of becoming infertile; indeed, some studies suggest that most women who have three or more attacks of PID become infertile. If the infection spreads from the tubes into the pelvic cavity it encourages the formation of strands of tissue called adhesions (see page 184), followed by scarring. Depending on its location, all this can produce various sorts of pain.

Nine times out of 10 PID results from a sexually transmitted infection. There's a 50:50 chance of chlamydia, gonorrhoea is next most likely and the two often co-exist. Unfortunately as many as 60 per cent women with chlamydia have no symptoms, so the infection often continues unchecked.

Other infecting organisms can enter the womb during a miscarriage; termination, sterilisation or other local surgery; or a womb examination or other gynae procedure. They occasionally enter during pregnancy (when they can encourage premature birth), during childbirth (especially in unhygienic conditions) or after childbirth (especially if part of the placenta doesn't come away).

Another cause is having a coil fitted when you have a vaginal infection; get it treated first or have tests and start antibiotics on the same day. One study found that the longer a woman had a coil the greater was her chance of pelvic infection. If you have a coil see your doctor for regular checks and at any time that you have a discharge, or unexpected bleeding or abdominal pain.

In seven out of 10 women with PID the cause is never discovered. Note that if a young girl has untreated threadworms (pinworms) it's possible, although extremely rare, for them to spread from her bowel via her vulva to the womb and cause PID.

what to do yourself

Change pads and tampons frequently – to help prevent infecting organisms from multiplying.

Rest – to help your immune system to deal with the infection. If you're in severe pain, lie on your back with your knees bent.

Dietary changes – Eat a healthy diet, including fresh garlic, and plenty of foods containing infection-fighting nutrients, such as beta-carotene, vitamins C and E, plant pigments, selenium and zinc. Also, drink enough to keep your urine very pale.

No smoking – This helps keep the circulation to your womb healthy. It also prevents the drain on your body's vitamin C, since your body uses 25mg of this vitamin to counteract the free radicals produced by inhaling the smoke from one cigarette.

Pelvic-floor and pelvic-tilt exercises – Do pelvic-floor exercises (see page 265) several times a day and pelvic-tilt exercies twice a day; kneeling on your hands and knees and rapidly rocking your lower back up and down for several minutes. These boost the pelvic circulation, which helps to fight infection.

Exercise – Take some 'whole-body' exercise (such as walking or swimming) each day (but not if you have a fever), as this boosts the circulation to your womb and encourages a good immune response.

Food supplements – It may be worth taking a supplement of vitamin C with flavonoids, especially if you continue to smoke. Other supplements that may be worth taking (though proof of their efficacy for PID is lacking) include beta-carotene, vitamin E, selenium and zinc.

Hydrotherapy – Stimulate your pelvic circulation with a daily contrast sitz bath (see page 275).

Heat / cold – Repeatedly apply alternate heat (from a hot-water bottle) and cold (from a covered freezer pack), for five minutes each to soothe the pain.

Painkillers – Take an over-the-counter painkiller, such as paracetamol or aspirin, if necessary (but only if you are sure your pain is due to PID, otherwise the pain relief might make you delay getting treatment for some other condition).

Herbal remedies – *Anemone pulsatilla* can help to relieve pain associated with inflammation and echinacea may help by boosting immunity. (Note the cautions on page 277 when using herbal remedies.

Ensure that your partner uses a condom until your PID is cured, because the risk of PID being caused by a sexually transmitted infection is so high. Even if there is no risk of your having such an infection a condom will protect your partner from the other infecting organisms you are harbouring.

Tests and investigations

Your doctor will take swabs from high in your vagina and send them to a laboratory to check the nature of the infecting organisms so as to determine the antibiotics most likely to work.

need to see a doctor?

Yes, because you need a diagnosis and antibiotics are vital to prevent infertility and repeated attacks. If your symptoms are severe you may need to stay in hospital.

It's particularly important to have a good test for chlamydia (the best probably being the polymerase chain reaction test, rather than the ELISA – enzyme-linked immunosorbent assay) because untreated chlamydia infection is particularly likely to cause serious complications such as infertility.

You need a pregnancy test if there's any chance that you might be pregnant because some first-choice antibiotics are unsuitable in pregnancy. Your sexual partner(s) is the most likely source of infection and should also, therefore, see a doctor.

If necessary, a gynaecologist will do a hysteroscopy and womb biopsy (or even laparoscopy) to confirm the diagnosis.

Medical treatment

Your doctor will prescribe antibiotics straight away, before the swab results are available. Some antibiotics may make the combined Pill less reliable, so make sure that your partner uses a condom or avoid sex until you've finished the course.

If continuing infection has damaged your fallopian tubes and you are having trouble getting pregnant, microsurgery via a laparoscope may be necessary to clear them. If the infection has spread from your tubes into your pelvis and caused adhesions and scar tissue around the pelvic organs, you may need laparoscopic surgery to free the organs.

your action plan

✔ Vital	✔ Could be vital	(✔) Optional
• Rest	• Exercise	• Food supplements
• Dietary changes		• Hydrotherapy
• No smoking		• Heat / cold
• Pelvic-tilt and pelvic- floor exercises		• Painkillers
• Medical treatment		• Herbal remedies

sex

Some of the most common problems involving a woman's sexual life include pain during sex and either a lack of sexual desire or the inability to become sexually aroused. Fortunately, there are many things you can do either alone or with your partner to help and, if necessary, you can consult your doctor or seek advice from a gynaecologist or psychosexual therapist.

painful sex

The first few times a woman has sex may hurt because of anxiety, being insufficiently aroused or having a tight vaginal entrance. Even women used to making love may find their vagina tightens when they're stressed, insufficiently aroused or tired or don't feel like sex for other reasons. Dryness can make sex painful and the scar from an episiotomy (a cut done to widen the vaginal opening and ease childbirth) may be uncomfortable for weeks or months. Painful sex may result from a vaginal infection, an inflamed cervix, a cervical erosion, irritated bladder or pelvic inflammatory disease. A vagina that's sensitive to condoms, spermicidal or lubricating creams or jellies can hurt during sex, as can an irritable bowel or a patch of endometriosis outside the

symptom sorter

Gynae or gynae-related causes of pain during sex

- ● ● ● **Most likely** – insufficient arousal, dry vulva and vagina, vagina-muscle spasm resulting from fear etc., vaginal infection

- ● ● **Less likely** – irritable bowel, endometriosis, stress, cystitis, sensitivity to condoms or spermicidal or lubricating products, cervical erosion, inflamed cervix, pelvic inflammatory disease

- ● **Possible** – recent episiotomy scar or vaginal tear during childbirth, cervix procedure or hysterectomy, over-long penis, fibroid or womb polyp stuck in the cervix, cervix polyp, ovary cyst, emotional 'scars' following a miscarriage, abortion or sexual abuse, prolapse, womb, ovary or cervix cancer

vagina. Sometimes an ovary cyst, a womb polyp or a fibroid stuck in the cervix, a cervix polyp, a prolapse or ovary or womb cancer are to blame. Occasionally sex is painful after a hysterectomy, possibly because of scar tissue at the top of the vagina.

Some women experience pain with one lover but not another and quite a lot of women who complain of painful sex have no discernible illness or pathology, yet their pain is very real. Sometimes deep-seated fear or other difficult emotions cause the vagina muscles to go into spasm. In such cases, women often benefit from counselling or psychosexual therapy as their pain may originate from mental, emotional or spiritual 'scars' from previous experiences such as abortion, miscarriage or sexual abuse.

what to do yourself

Relax, take time over foreplay and use a vaginal lubricant unless you are sensitive to this. Identify and treat the underlying cause. Talk the problem over with your partner and see if you can come up with some answers yourselves.

Tests and investigations

Whether or not anything other than a simple physical examination is required depends on the circumstances.

Medical treatment

This depends on the cause. For example, for postmenopausal dryness of the vulva and vagina your doctor might recommend oestrogen cream, and for pelvic inflammatory disease, antibiotics.

need to see a doctor?

Yes, if the discomfort is severe or if it continues and is unexplained. You may need help from a counsellor or even a psychosexual therapist for stress, causes that lie in your past or relationship-related discomfort.

your action plan

✔ **Could be vital**

• Medical assessment

• Home treatments (see What to do yourself, above)

• Medical treatment

low sex drive or arousal

If you are feeling 'off' sex you may still be having it because your partner wants it, or because it's a habit, but you're less likely to initiate sexual activity, have sexy dreams or daydreams, or climax with your partner or on your own. Does it matter? The answer is 'yes', because you could be missing out unnecessarily and your partner is missing out on having a partner who fancies him. Research also suggests that an active sex life sometimes prolongs life. If there's nothing wrong with your sex drive but you no longer want sex with your partner, there may be a chance of rekindling the spark you once had.

Many factors can reduce your sex drive or sexual response.

Physical causes – Probably the most common cause is the man or the woman not spending long enough over her arousal or not being skilled enough. Another possibility is insufficient opportunity for sex, as many people find the more they have sex, the more they want it. Feeling tired is a common culprit – especially in women who have a young baby or are trying to work *and* be a mother, housewife and lover. Some women go off sex before a period, others when pregnant, breastfeeding or menopausal. Environmental discomfort such as being too hot or cold can be a turn-off. Overindulgence in alcohol is a possibility, as are certain drugs (such as beta-blockers for high blood pressure and some antidepressants). A hormone deficiency (such as too little testosterone – due to the body producing less testosterone when stressed but more of a stress hormone called cortisol) and ageing are also possibilities. (However, age isn't often a barrier to interest in sex; one study, for example, found that four in five married women aged 70-79 were sexually active.) Older women (and men) may take longer to become aroused and need to use more patience, good humour, expertise and inventiveness; also, intercourse itself may become less important than other sources of sexual and sensual pleasure. Sometimes hidden or known illness is to blame for a lack of interest in sex – possibilities include an underactive thyroid, arterial disease, diabetes, anorexia nervosa, a high prolactin level (see 'Nipple itching and/or discharge, page 70), and anything that causes pain.

Psychological causes – You may go off sex when you feel stressed or upset, or if you have relationship problems, are depressed or fear getting, or not getting, pregnant. Another possibility is fear of anything to do with your genitals, perhaps after a difficult labour or genital surgery. Some women fear criticism of their body, sexuality or sexual technique, losing control, being hurt or being overheard or otherwise discovered. Your man may no longer turn you on because he isn't loving and affectionate or has become a bully or gone to seed. It's perfectly possible to feel loving toward your partner but not fancy him. Other women consciously or unconsciously perceive their man as a parent figure rather than a lover. Some women have problems because they identify with their mother whom they consider sexless or because they can't fantasise and, if they do, they can imagine sex only with someone other than their partner; guilt can be a real turn-off. Some women may have been conditioned as children to believe it's wrong to express their sexuality. Finally, in some women sex brings up conscious or unconscious memories of sexual abuse.

what to do yourself

Attend to the cause – Try to identify what's to blame and attend to it if possible. If you don't know, talking things through with your partner may help. It's also wise to boost your general health so as to encourage healthy hormone levels.

Get aroused – Use as much patience, humour, expertise, creativity and ingenuity, as you need to become aroused. If necessary, use a lubricant (such as saliva, or a commercial product such as KY jelly) to prevent discomfort.

No smoking – This is very wise, since smoking can damage arteries and reduce the blood flow to the various parts of your body involved in sex drive and sexual response. These include the brain, pituitary, hypothalamus, adrenal glands, ovaries and clitoris.

Exercise – Take regular aerobic exercise to boost your circulation and encourage healthy hormone levels.

Pelvic floor exercises (see page 265) – Do several batches of these a day to boost pelvic circulation, tone pelvic-floor muscles and increase vaginal moisture production. All this may encourage sexual arousal and increase your pleasure from orgasm and sex.

symptom sorter

Gynae or gynae-related causes of low sex drive/arousal

● ● ● **Most likely** – relationship problems, insufficient arousal, insufficient opportunity for sex, fatigue, oestrogen deficiency, hormone changes (premenstrual, menopausal, or associated with pregnancy or breastfeeding), environmental discomfort, too much alcohol, stress, fear of getting or not getting pregnant, no fanciable partner, guilt during an affair

● ● **Less likely** – fear of criticism, losing control, being hurt, or being discovered; guilt or shame about sex; too little testosterone; inability to fantasise; ageing; certain drugs; pain; illness; fear of contracting or passing on a sexually transmitted infection

● **Possible** – depression, fear after a difficult labour or genital surgery, perception of partner as a parent figure, identification with 'sexless' mother, conscious or unconscious memories of sexual abuse, high prolactin level

Exposure to light – Getting enough bright outdoor daylight on your skin, and in your eyes, boosts your production of sex hormones, and of 'feel-good' endorphins and serotonin (see page 16), which may make you feel more interested in sex. If you get winter depression, consider using a light visor or box.

Dietary changes – Eat more foods rich in vitamins B and E, zinc and plant oestrogens. Include brown rice and foods made from whole rye or wheat grains, as these contain an amino acid called histidine, said to aid sexual arousal. The balance of two amino acids, arginine and lysine, may affect your sex drive (since arginine can boost the circulation as long as you don't have too much lysine), so try eating more arginine-rich food (nuts, beans, seeds, cereal-grain foods, even chocolate – though only in moderation, perhaps a small bar each day if this fits into a healthy diet) and less lysine-rich food (fish, eggs, meat, milk, yoghurt, potatoes, beans, bean sprouts).

Healthy weight maintenance – You'll probably feel better about your body image, more interested in sex and more sexually attractive, if you keep within the weight range that's right for your build.

Stress management – Find effective ways of managing life's inevitable stresses. Remember, though, that even if you don't feel like sex, you may become more interested once you start. Sex can be an excellent stress-buster.

Mind techniques – Take time to identify your emotions about sex and try to establish where they originate. If they are putting you off sex, find ways of dealing with them. Sometimes simply naming difficult emotions prevents them becoming a barrier to good sex. Some women benefit greatly from learning the skills needed to manage anger and conflict.

Food supplements – Experiment to see if taking a regular multivitamin and mineral supplement helps.

Massage and aromatherapy – Having a 'sensual' massage or giving one to your partner can be an excellent way of boosting sexual interest, especially if sex has become too mechanical and predictable so that it's a rush to have sex rather than 'make love'. Lubricating the skin with scented oil enhances a massage. Ylang ylang, rose, ginger and sandalwood oils are particularly good ones to try – choose any two and add three drops of each to two teaspoons of sweet almond or other carrier oil.

 Relaxing in a scented bath before sex, or bathing with your partner, could help you to wind down after a busy day. Choose any two of the above oils, and put three drops of each in your bath water (though if you are using ginger oil, add it to a tablespoon of carrier oil first, or it could irritate your skin).

Hydrotherapy, heat and cold – Try a contrast sitz bath (see page 275) before sex to stimulate your pelvic circulation, or shower with alternately comfortably hot, then cool water.

Herbal remedies – Herbs might be worth trying. *Vitex agnus castus,* dong quai, *Muira puama,* catuaba, ginseng and astragalus help some women. When in one study 80 postmenopausal women took *agnus castus,* many felt more interested in sex. This is ironic because this herb is also called chasteberry and – because it reduces sex drive in men – monk's pepper but herbalists have always claimed it does makes women feel more sexy. (Note the advice on page 277, when using herbal remedies.)

Relationship therapy – If you've lost interest in lovemaking for emotional or relationship reasons, consider seeing a counsellor or psychosexual therapist yourself, or having couple counselling.

Be philosophical – Take comfort that things may change. Try mutual masturbation. Enjoy other sensual pleasures such as a shoulder rub, cuddling or hugging your nearest and dearest, stroking a pet, wearing silk next to your skin and appreciating the beauty of nature and music. Express passion and creativity in other ways such as painting, creative writing, dancing, researching your family tree, becoming involved in local politics, playing an instrument, or joining a singing group, or a book club or other discussion group. The main thing is not to allow feeling off sex to become a major crisis in your relationship. Agree, perhaps, not to have sex for, say, a month and do lots of other loving things together as in your courtship days. Lastly, remember that millions of couples of all ages are happy together even though they hardly ever have sex.

Tests and investigations

Your doctor will examine you, if necessary and do any investigations required to rule out physical causes. You may, for example, need a urine test for diabetes or a blood test for an underactive thyroid. If you are on any medications, your doctor can tell you whether these could be to blame.

need to see a doctor?

Yes, if none of the above works because your doctor can help you to work out the cause and address it.

Medical treatment

This depends on the cause. For example, if sex hurts, your vagina could be tensing and drying up because you're stressed or tired. Alternatively, scarring after childbirth or a hysterectomy may be the culprit. You may have an infection or be sensitive to condoms or spermicidal or lubricating creams or jellies. Or there may be a loop of irritable bowel or a patch of endometriosis outside your vagina. Your doctor will suggest treatment if necessary. Some women who've had their menopause find HRT patches useful though oral HRT doesn't help.

While the drug sildenafil (Viagra) was not licensed for women at the time of writing, a recent study found that women who took it had more intercourse and orgasms, possibly because it increased the blood flow to their genitals, including the clitoris.

your action plan

✔ **Vital**	✔ **Could be vital**	(✔) **Optional**
• Attend to the cause	• Dietary changes	• Food supplements
• Get aroused	• Healthy weight	• Massage and
• No smoking	maintenance	aromatherapy
• Exercise	• Stress management	• Hydrotherapy, heat and
• Exposure to light	• Mind techniques	cold
	• Medical treatment	• Herbal remedies
	• Relationship therapy	
	• Be philosophical	

sexually transmitted infections

The most likely infections are due to yeast-like fungi (candida), one-celled organisms called protozoa (*Trichomonas vaginalis*), bacteria (gonococci, and syphilis spirochaetes), bacteria-like organisms (*Chlamydia trachomatis)* and viruses (*Herpes simplex* or HSV, human papillomaviruses or HPV and human immunodeficiency viruses or HIV). Syphilis can be identified by a blood test but isn't covered here, as it's very much less common than the other infections.

A sexually transmitted infection may cause a vaginal discharge and/or soreness, pelvic pain, and a fever, although some infections, such as chlamydia and gonorrhoea, can be 'silent' for some time. Some infections can lead to serious problems such as infertility or cancer, and HIV can lead to AIDS (autoimmune deficiency syndrome).

what to do yourself

General anti-STI measures

Safer sex

• The only sure way of preventing these infections is for you and your partner to be infection-free at the beginning of your sexual relationship and to be faithful to each other.

• If this is impossible or undesirable always ensure that your partner uses a condom when you have sex, even if you are on the Pill.

• Be alert to symptoms if you think your sex life, or your partner's, puts you at risk.

• If your partner has an infection either avoid sex or be sure that he uses a condom and gets treated (and get yourself checked too).

• If you have an infection either avoid sex until the infection is cured or protect your partner by ensuring that he uses a condom, or by wearing a female condom yourself (or, for oral sex, a square of thin latex rubber known as a dental dam).

• If you are infected tell your partner so that he can be tested and, if infected, get treated and, meanwhile, use a condom.

• Be aware that you are less resistant in the few days before a period because premenstrual hormone changes reduce immunity and make genital moisture less protective.

• Be aware that infections can be passed on by vaginal, oral and anal sex, by sharing sex toys, by touching each other's genitals and your own, and, for lesbians, by rubbing vulvas together.

Dietary changes – Boost your immunity by eating a healthy diet with plenty of foods rich in beta-carotene, vitamins C and E, folic acid, flavonoid plant pigments (especially proanthocyanidins), selenium and zinc and eat more foods rich in omega-3 fatty acids and less food rich in omega-6s. Also, use two raw garlic cloves each day – for example, in salad dressings.

No smoking – as cigarette smoke in the body reduces immunity. It's also wise to avoid passive smoking.

Pelvic floor exercises (see page 265) – Doing these several times a day boosts the circulation in your pelvis, which may aid recovery.

Stress management – Find effective ways of managing the inevitable stresses in life – including the stress of having an STI – as continuing stress dampens immunity.

Exercise – A daily half hour of gentle-to-moderate, whole-body exercise may help by boosting your immunity, and increasing the circulation to your pelvis.

Food supplements – Consider aiming to boost your immunity further by taking supplements of beta-carotene, vitamins C and E, flavonoids (including proanthocyanidins), folic acid, selenium and zinc.

Tests and investigations

You need swabs to reveal the type of infection and to determine appropriate treatment – with suitable antibiotics, for example, for bacterial infections.

need to see a doctor?

Go to your doctor or to a genito-urinary medicine (GUM) clinic without delay if you suspect a sexually transmitted infection. Your partner and any other sexual contacts should also be seen and treated if necessary.

your action plan

✔ Vital

- Medical treatment
- Safer sex
- Dietary changes

- No smoking
- Pelvic floor exercises
- Stress management

✔ Could be vital

- Exercise

(✔) Optional

- Food supplements

chlamydia infection

Bacteria-like organisms called *Chlamydia trachomatis* can be transmitted during sex and to a baby during childbirth. Chlamydia infection is on the increase and is now the most common treatable sexually transmitted disease in Europe and many other countries. Many countries have seen an alarming rise in chlamydia infection in teenagers because of the tendency to have sex younger and to have more sexual partners. In the UK it affects almost one in 10 sexually active women under 25.

Around seven in ten women with chlamydia have no warning signs, as the infection is often 'silent' – meaning free from the initial symptoms of infection – with the organisms hiding unnoticed in the cervix, womb, fallopian tubes, or bladder. Indeed, between three and fourteen women in every hundred who attend family planning clinics are infected, yet between 50 and 70 per cent of them experience no symptoms. When chlamydia does make itself known early on, it's usually with some combination of vaginal inflammation, a discharge that's likely to be yellowish, low abdominal and/or pelvic pain, bleeding between periods or after sex, fever, pain during sex and pain on passing urine. Some people also get conjunctivitis ('pink eye'). However, these initial symptoms may not show up until one to three weeks or even as long as several months after infection.

One concern is that untreated infection can spread to your womb and fallopian tubes, causing pelvic inflammatory disease and making the tubes inflamed and scarred. If you become pregnant this raises the risk of a miscarriage or ectopic pregnancy (one outside the womb). Most important, it also raises the risk of infertility. If your cervix is also infected with human papillomaviruses (HPV, see page 204), it encourages cervix cancer too.

what to do yourself

A home kit to test your urine for chlamydia is available, but relatively expensive (see Helplist, page 315).

Take general anti-STI measures – see page 199

Be wary of having a 'coil' fitted – if you have a chlamydia infection involving your cervix this could push the infection into the womb and encourage pelvic inflammatory disease. Either wait or start antibiotics at once.

Tests and investigations

If your symptoms and/or an examination suggest chlamydia infection, the doctor will arrange tests on your urine, tampons, or swabs from your vulva or cervix, to check whether chlamydia is the culprit. The newest tests are claimed to have a 90 per cent success rate. If you have chlamydia your partner(s) will need checking too and treating, if necessary; note that in one in two men with chlamydia the infection is 'silent'.

Medical treatment

This is with antibiotics.

need to see a doctor?

Yes, go to your doctor – or a genito-urinary medicine (GUM) clinic – without delay if you are experiencing symptoms or even if you are not but your risk is high and you suspect you might have a 'silent' infection. This is because chlamydia infection is treatable with antibiotics and the earlier it's tested for, and treated, the better. Tests are positive a few days after infection, even if you are symptom free. There's currently no plan in the UK to routinely screen all women at high risk of chlamydia infection but researchers are assessing whether more women should be offered screening tests. If so, they'll probably be offered to sexually active under-25s, older women with two or more partners in the last 12 months, women undergoing a termination, pregnant women, those attending GUM clinics and, perhaps, those about to have a coil fitted.

your action plan

✔ **Vital**

- Medical treatment
- General anti-STI measures (see page 199)
- Avoid having a coil fitted

gonorrhoea

This is a sexually transmitted disease caused by infection with bacteria called *Neisseria gonorhoea* (gonococci). The infection usually involves the cervix but can affect the urethra (the urine passage between bladder and vulva), rectum, throat and conjunctiva (the layer of cells covering eyes and lining lids). The time from infection to the start of symptoms is usually 2-10 days but can be as long as three weeks.

The infection is 'silent' in up to seven women in 10. However, possible symptoms include a vaginal discharge (which comes from inflamed cervix cells), pelvic pain, pain on passing water, pain in the rectum, a repeated unsuccessful urge to open the bowels and mucus, blood or pus in the stools. Other possibilities include conjunctivitis ('pink eye') and a sore throat. If left untreated, it may inflame the Bartholin's glands in the vulva (page 167) and spread to the fallopian tubes, causing infertility. At worst, it can cause blood poisoning (septicaemia) with a rash and arthritis.

what to do yourself

Take general STI measures – see page 199

Tests and investigations

Your doctor will take swabs from your cervix and send them to a laboratory without delay, as they spoil quickly. The lab will confirm the cause of the infection, and test to see which antibiotics are suitable.

need to see a doctor?

Yes, but it's best go to a doctor at a genito-urinary medicine (GUM) clinic. Your partner(s) should see a doctor too.

Medical treatment

Your doctor will recommend starting antibiotics immediately after the swabs are taken; you can always change to another type of antibiotic if the swab results suggest this would be more helpful. The doctor may also recommend treatment for chlamydia infection at the same time as this is so common in women with gonorrhoea.

your action plan

✔ **Vital**

• Medical treatment

• General anti-STI measures (see page 199)

hpv infection

There are over 80 types of human papillomavirus (HPV, or wart virus). Sexually transmitted infection with certain types can cause warts on the vulva, around the back passage, in the vagina or rectum, on the cervix and, rarely, in the mouth and throat. It can also cause a 'silent' infection of the vulva or cervix – one that you cannot see and does not cause symptoms – and it can help to trigger cancer of the vulva or cervix.

Genital warts – generally caused by HPV types 6 and 11 – are single or multiple, flat or cauliflower-shaped, and may have a stalk. They are most common in women in their 20s. The first signs may appear two to four weeks after the infection begins, or they may not show for several months. The infected sites feel itchy and you may notice a burning feeling; later warts may appear.

Infection of the cervix or vulva encourages pre-cancerous cells to develop, though this is generally a possibility only with HPV types 16 and 18 (and, to a lesser extent, 31, 33 and 35). These 'high-risk' or 'oncogenic' (cancer-encouraging) types are less likely to cause warts. Type 16 is most likely to persist in the cervix and is most commonly found in cervix cancer. Untreated, infection of the cervix or vulva with high-risk types may cause cancer.

The viruses need moisture to survive and experts disagree as to whether hands or towels can transfer viruses.

what to do yourself

Take general anti-STI measures (see page 199) – Also, be aware that oral sex with an infected person is highly likely to transmit the viruses.

Other dietary changes – The balance of two amino acids, arginine and lysine, may affect your susceptibility to viral infection, so eat more lysine-rich foods (fish, eggs, meat, milk, yoghurt, potatoes, beans – especially bean sprouts) and cut down on arginine (in nuts, seeds, cereal grains, chocolate).

Tests and investigations

A doctor can check for the likelihood of invisible infection by painting the area with dilute acetic acid, which whitens infected cells more deeply and for longer than it does normal ones. Tests for HPV will be arranged if necessary. It's also wise to have a cervical smear.

need to see a doctor?

See your family doctor, if necessary, before going to a gynaecologist or genito-urinary medicine (GUM) doctor. Be aware that you may have other sexually transmitted infections. If you get a sudden crop of genital warts, see your doctor without delay, as your immunity could be suppressed by an illness such as HIV infection. Your sexual partner(s) should see a doctor too.

Medical treatment

Warts on the vulva or around the anus can be treated with cream containing imiquimod (which alters the local immune response) or repeated applications of podophyllum solution or cream (protecting surrounding skin with petroleum jelly – or Vaseline). Researchers are investigating the possibility of treating the cervix with imiquimod.

In some cases warts need to be numbed, then frozen (with liquid nitrogen) or zapped with a laser. Cervical warts are usually lasered.

your action plan

✔ **Vital**

- Medical treatment
- General anti-STI measures
  (see page 199)

✔ **Could be vital**

- Other dietary changes

hepatitis b and c

Infection of the liver with hepatitis B or C viruses, or other hepatitis viruses, makes the liver inflamed; viral infection is by far the commonest cause of hepatitis. Hepatitis B is caught from infected blood, saliva, semen, urine, or faeces; hepatitis C mainly from infected blood. Having unprotected sex with someone who knowingly or unknowingly has hepatitis puts you at high risk of catching it. Other people with a high risk of hepatitis B and C include those who have previously had a sexually transmitted infection, drug users who share needles, those who share a toothbrush or razor with an infected person and those who have tattoos, body piercing, or acupuncture done with unsterilised equipment. An infected woman can infect her baby during pregnancy or birth and health workers can also succumb by pricking themselves with an infected needle or getting infected blood on a break in their skin, such as a sore or a cut on the hand.

One to six months after becoming infected with hepatitis B or C viruses, you may get a flu-like illness, followed by nausea, vomiting, diarrhoea, abdominal pain, jaundice (yellow skin and dark urine), itching and extreme fatigue. Two in three people with hepatitis B have no symptoms or only mild ones, though; and nine in 10 people with hepatitis C have none.

Hepatitis B and C are highly contagious for up to three months after the initial illness. Acute hepatitis is usually over in four to eight weeks, though you may feel exhausted for months. However, in up to one person in 10 with hepatitis B and up to one in two of those with hepatitis C, the liver becomes chronically inflamed.

Symptoms can rumble on for years, the condition remains infectious and the infection may gradually – perhaps over several decades – damage the liver, causing cirrhosis (scarring and hardening), liver failure, or even cancer.

what to do yourself

To prevent hepatitis B and C, avoid casual unprotected sex or sex with anyone who you know to have hepatitis. No one knows for sure whether hepatitis viruses can be caught by oral sex. However, it is likely, especially if you have a cut or sore in your mouth, lips, vulva, vagina or cervix (or, if you have anal sex, a cut or sore in your back passage or rectum). Also, avoid tattoos, body piercing, or acupuncture unless done with sterilised equipment. IV-drug users should not share needles. Hepatitis B immunisation helps to protect high-risk people.

Take general STI measures – see page 199

Other dietary changes – Have a healthy light diet, with plenty of water but no alcohol, so you give your liver as little work as possible.

No medications – Don't take any medication without your doctor's approval in order to protect your delicate liver from the work of breaking it down.

Rest – Take as much rest as you need to cope with fatigue and weakness.

Food supplements – Some people benefit from supplements of vitamin B, C and E, selenium, and an anti-oxidant called alpha-lipoic acid. But discuss this with your doctor first.

Herbal remedies – Some people benefit from milk thistle (silymarin) but discuss this with your doctor before taking it.

Tests and investigations

Blood tests and, perhaps, a liver biopsy (a sample taken with a needle passed into the liver through the abdomen) clinch the diagnosis. Routine blood tests reveal hepatitis B in pregnant women, enabling immunisation of their babies after birth and treatment for them.

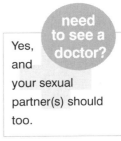

need to see a doctor?

Yes, and your sexual partner(s) should too.

Medical treatment

There's no specific treatment for acute hepatitis, though a few people need hospital care. The good news is that treatment with interferon or lamivudine for chronic hepatitis B, and interferon and, perhaps, ribavirin for chronic hepatitis C, encourages permanent recovery.

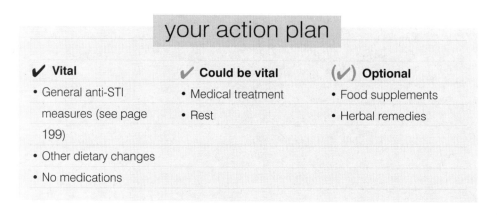

your action plan

✔ **Vital**	✔ **Could be vital**	(✔) **Optional**
• General anti-STI measures (see page 199)	• Medical treatment	• Food supplements
	• Rest	• Herbal remedies
• Other dietary changes		
• No medications		

herpes infection

Herpes simplex virus (HSV) infection can cause lip sores (cold sores). It can also affect other areas of skin; the vulva, vagina and cervix (when it's called genital herpes); the back passage; the throat and (usually only in young babies) the eyes and brain.

Sexually transmitted herpes is the commonest cause of genital ulcers. This most often results from a different strain of herpes virus (HSV type 2) from the one that causes cold sores and is usually caught from sex with a partner with genital herpes. However, HSV type 1 viruses – the ones that generally cause cold sores – are increasingly likely to be responsible for genital infection. Indeed, one in two new, severe, genital infections are due to HSV1. The HSV2 viruses generally cause only genital symptoms.

Genital herpes is very common and relatively harmless. Most women have been infected with HSV1 for the first time by the age of 25 and studies suggest that in the UK, one in eight women has been infected with HSV2. Herpes infection is permanent but generally lies dormant most or all of the time.

Genital herpes infection is caught by contact between a break in your skin and someone else's infected sore. During a first attack blisters erupt on your vulva (and, perhaps, vagina, cervix, buttocks and thighs) within seven days, then form small but very painful ulcers that eventually heal. Sores in your vulva may make passing urine very painful. The first infection usually causes fever, fatigue and headaches, with joint and muscle pain and swollen lymph nodes ('glands'). The viruses then travel along the nerves that supply the infected site and 'hibernate' near the spinal cord. Once there certain triggers can reactivate symptoms; these include stress, periods, infections, skin damage and fatigue. One person in two with a long-term herpes infection has recurrent sores, characterised by tingling, itching or stinging.

Many women never notice another attack, though recurrences are more likely with HSV2 infections or if the primary attack was severe. Reactivated infection generally produces only mild symptoms, including soreness and pain on passing urine and is much more likely with HSV2 infection. So if you think you've caught genital herpes from someone with a cold sore, the odds are it will be less likely to recur. Most people have four to six recurrences a year but recurrences are more likely in the first six months.

what to do yourself

Avoid triggers – Steer clear of anything you know triggers recurrent infections.

Take general anti-STI measures – see page 199.

Other dietary changes – Eat two raw garlic cloves each day. The balance of two amino acids, arginine and lysine, may affect your susceptibility to viral infection so eat more lysine-rich foods (fish, shellfish, eggs, meat, milk, yoghurt, beans, bean sprouts, potatoes), and cut down on arginine (in nuts, seeds, cereal grains, corn, rice, chocolate).

Safe sex – If you have sores, or think you're about to get them because of the familiar premonitory tingling, itching or stinging on your lip, vulva or elsewhere, avoid sex and return to it only when they are completely healed. Use condoms between times, even when the infection is quiet, since there is a small risk of passing on infection when you are well.

If you have a cold sore, don't kiss anyone (especially if they are very young, unwell or pregnant, or have widespread eczema) or perform oral sex on your partner (even with a condom, or dam – a thin sheet of rubber over your vulva – since these give scant protection).

Skin care – Avoid touching a cold sore or genital sore. If you do touch it, wash your hands well and dry them thoroughly on kitchen paper, or a towel you keep to yourself and launder at as high a temperature as possible. Cold sores usually heal better if kept moist and covered with a layer of fats to reduce their contact with air. Achieve this with frequent applications (with a cotton bud) of any ointment, cream or oil, applied when the tingling starts. Particularly useful remedies include lavender and tea tree oils and vitamin A and E oils (obtained by piercing a vitamin A or E capsule). To make a useful cream for herpes sores on lips or genitals, buy 30g of unscented cold cream and add nine drops of lavender or rose oil and six of tea tree oil. Or use melissa ointment (see below). Some people prefer to treat a cold sore with surgical spirit or witch hazel – or even black coffee. Over-the-counter remedies for cold sores include ingredients such as iodine, menthol, ammonia, phenol and alcohol.

Take painkillers – Over-the-counter painkillers, such as paracetamol, may be vital for painful genital sores.

Hydrotherapy – Soothe pain from genital herpes sores by applying a cool compress or a compress containing moist bicarbonate of soda (baking soda), or by having a salt bath (put a small handful of salt in the bath water and stir). If urination is very painful you may find that urinating while you are lying in bath water is more comfortable.

Food supplements – Consider taking vitamin C with flavonoids, zinc, and lysine, to help combat the infection.

Herbal remedies – Take a teaspoon of echinacea tincture in a little water twice a day by mouth for two months to boost immunity. Smooth melissa (lemon balm) ointment (see Helplist, page 315) on sores twice a day. (Note the cautions on page 277 when using herbal remedies.)

Tests and investigations

Blood tests and tests of genital swabs by a laboratory identify genital herpes infection. If positive you have a raised risk of other sexually transmitted infections, so your doctor may do tests for these. Your partner(s) should also be checked.

need to see a doctor?

Yes, if you suspect genital herpes. If it's your first attack it's best to go to a genitourinary medicine (GUM) clinic. This is also wise if you get six or more attacks a year, as you may need long-term antiviral treatment.

Medical treatment

For first attacks of genital herpes, or for troublesome recurrences, you will probably need oral antiviral drugs (such as aciclovir, valaciclovir, and famciclovir) for five days, perhaps starting before the test results are available. Such drugs are worthwhile if begun up to six days after the start of symptoms, or if you still have blisters on your vulva, as they reduce pain, clear up symptoms and shorten the time that you are infectious. Cream containing an antiviral drug doesn't help the first attack. However, a prescription for aciclovir cream is useful so that if you get another attack of herpes blisters in your vulva you can use it straight away.

If you are pregnant there's a tiny risk that any genital sores present at the time of giving birth could infect your baby, so your doctor will check before delivery. If you have active genital herpes you may be advised to have a caesarean section.

your action plan

✔ **Vital**	✔ **Could be vital**	(✔) **Optional**
• Avoiding triggers	• Medical treatment	• Food supplements
• General anti-STI measures (see page 199)	• Painkillers	• Herbal remedies
	• Other dietary changes	
• Safe sex	• Hydrotherapy	
• Skin care		

trichomonas infection

Sexually transmitted infection with the bacteria-like organisms called *Trichomonas vaginalis* may cause no symptoms, although it sometimes leads to itching of the vagina and vulva, a yellowish–green, frothy vaginal discharge that may smell fishy, and abdominal pain. In a pregnant woman it can encourage premature labour and make her baby more likely to have a low birth weight.

what to do yourself

Take general anti-STI measures – see page 199.

Herbal remedies – Consider taking beth root and echinacea and bathing your vulva with goldenseal tea. (Note the cautions on page 277, when using herbal remedies.)

Tests and investigations

These may include examining a sample of any discharge under a microscope, measuring the degree of acidity (pH) in the vagina (which is raised with this infection) and sending vaginal swabs to a laboratory for identification of the infection.

Yes.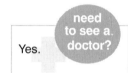

Medical treatment

This is with a drug called metronidazole. Your partner(s) should also have treatment.

your action plan

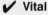 **Vital**

- Medical treatment
- General anti-STI measures (see page 199)

hiv infection and aids

Infection with human immunodeficiency viruses (HIV) is a growing problem in most countries and a national tragedy in some African countries where it kills many people. It generally infects people via semen, blood or cervical secretions during unprotected sex with an infected person – though virus-carrying body fluid requires contact with broken skin or mucous membrane in the other person for the viruses to enter their body. Anal intercourse is particularly risky, partly because the anal lining is readily damaged. A drug called amyl nitrate (sold as 'poppers' and used to relax the anus) is suspected of encouraging infection. A woman infected with HIV can pass it to her unborn or breastfeeding child. Infection can also be spread by infected donated blood, body organs or semen; contaminated needles; razors or toothbrushes, although this risk is small; and 'needlestick injuries' (via a prick with a contaminated needle).

HIV infection gradually depresses the immune system, leading to a variety of health problems. It initially shows up in 25-65 per cent of affected people as a mild glandular-fever-like illness, perhaps with candida infection in the mouth; occasionally, there are more severe symptoms, such as meningitis. The next stage is symptom free and lasts up to 10 years. The third stage may involve swelling of lymph nodes ('glands') around the body, persisting for around three months. Autoimmune deficiency syndrome, or AIDS, is the last, and fatal stage. It involves the reactivation of viruses that have been relatively 'silent' and can show as a general illness (such as a fever, sweating, weight loss and diarrhoea) and problems with the skin, mouth and blood.

what to do yourself

Take general anti-STI measures – see page 199.

Other safer-sex tips – If you perform oral sex on a man who has (or you think might have) HIV infection, without him using a condom, at least ensure that he doesn't ejaculate in your mouth. This is even more important if his penis and/or your mouth is sore. Alternatively, reduce your risk by spitting out his semen at once, or swallow it (since stomach acid inactivates HIV), then rinse your mouth well with water. If he wants to do oral sex on you, refuse if he has mouth ulcers, gum disease, or thrush or if you have a sore vulva. Be aware that neither male nor female condoms give 100 per cent protection.

Other exercise tips – Avoid over-exertion as this depresses immunity.

Other dietary tips – Aim to be some pounds heavier than the average normal weight for your height (but avoid obesity). Eat full-fat dairy foods rather than lower-fat ones, as the vitamins (A and D) in their fats are useful and be sure to eat enough foods containing selenium and quercetin (a flavonoid in onions, apple peel, cabbage, tea and red wine), both of which have antiviral activity.

Herbal remedies – One herb that shows promise against HIV in the test tube is box, whose effect seems to mimic that of AZT (see Medical treatment, below); however, under no circumstances should you self-prescribe this herb as it is poisonous. Other potentially useful herbs include damask rose, which has moderate anti-HIV activity in the test tube, and a type of chrysanthemum (*Chrysanthemum morifolium*). If you want to try herbal remedies for HIV infection, only do so with the guidance of a fully qualified herbalist. Also note the cautions on page 277 when using herbal remedies.

Tests and investigations

You need blood tests to confirm the presence of HIV and to test for other sexually transmitted infections.

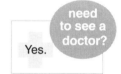
Yes. need to see a doctor?

Medical treatment

There is considerable interest in aiming to recognise the initial infection and give drugs called retroviral agents (such as zidovudine, or AZT) within 12-18 months of this, as these may delay or even prevent HIV infection from developing into AIDS. A drug called interleukin can help to improve immunity. The same agents can be helpful during the later stages too. The big hope at present is for an effective vaccine.

your action plan

✔ Vital

- Medical treatment
- General anti-STI measures (see page 199)

- Other safer-sex tips
- Other exercise tips

✔ Could be vital

- Other dietary tips

menopause

Your last period is symbolically important as it marks the end of your natural reproductive life. However, it can also mark the beginning of new opportunities, and perhaps, given that any children are likely to be grown up, more time for other interests.

hot flushes, night sweats and other menopausal signs

Four out of five women in westernised countries experience hot flushes around the menopause. These sudden waves of uncontrollable blushing and warmth over the face, neck, and sometimes the chest, last from several seconds to several minutes and may occur many times a day. They are thought to result from falling levels of oestrogen and, perhaps, progesterone, stimulating surges of luteinising hormone which make small blood vessels over-sensitive and prone to sudden dilation. They usually stop within two or three years, though they can continue for up to five years in one in four women and indefinitely in one in 20. They may also cause bouts of sweating at night. Flushes and sweats also occur in women who come off HRT too quickly. Most women don't mind flushes; some see them as a badge of maturity and the 'change of life', and a symbol of wisdom; others find they interfere with their work, social life, and sleep.

In Japanese women living in Japan, flushes are virtually unknown, which researchers suggest is because their traditional diet is rich in soy protein (from soy beans and tofu) and therefore in plant oestrogens.

Unusual breast tenderness and, perhaps, lumpiness can result from changing hormone levels. Some women also report depression and, while this could result from the lifestyle changes that often occur at this time, it's been pointed out that the surges in luteinising hormone that are common around the menopause can trigger surges in 'feel-good' hormone-like substances called endorphins and that falling endorphin levels after such surges could trigger depression.

A low oestrogen level encourages a dry vulva and vagina and may reduce libido. Some women also report fatigue, dry skin, poor concentration and memory, headaches, aching muscles and joints, dull hair and brittle nails, though whether these symptoms are oestrogen-related is unclear.

Some months or years after the menopause, some women develop cystitis-like symptoms (see urethral syndrome, page 174) associated with thinning of the lining of the lining of the urethra due to a low oestrogen level. Their risk of osteoporosis gradually rises, too.

what to do yourself

Troublesome flushes and sweats nearly always go eventually but you can help them on their way.

Exercise – Take a daily half hour of moderately vigorous exercise to help keep your blood vessels in good condition.

Stress management – Use effective stress management since high levels of stress hormones worsen flushes and sweats.

symptom sorter

Gynae or gynae-related causes of hot flushes and night sweats

- ● ● ● **Most likely** – menopause, rosacea
- ● ● **Less likely** – 'stress', blushing from embarrassment, oversensitivity to hot drinks or food
- ● **Possible** – certain drugs, overactive thyroid; carcinoid (serotonin-producing tumour of the gut, ovary or lung), phaeochromocytoma (an adrenal tumour producing, for example, adrenaline)

Exposure to light – Go outside in bright daylight each day to boost oestrogen production and reduce any rapid falls in its level.

Dietary changes – Eat more foods rich in plant oestrogens. Also, try coriander tea, made by soaking two tablespoons of coriander seeds in a cup of cold water overnight, then straining – and warming if desired – before drinking.

Hydrotherapy – Each day, take a comfortably hot shower, then turn the water temperature to cool or even cold for 10 seconds or so, to stimulate your circulation and help keep blood vessels healthy.

Aromatherapy massage – Ask someone to give you a whole-body, hand, foot, shoulder or face massage. Or massage your own legs, arms or abdomen. Lubricate the skin with three drops of lavender or ylang ylang (to aid relaxation), and three drops of rose, clary sage, geranium or fennel oils (to help prevent rapid hormone fluctuations) in two tablespoons of sweet almond (or other carrier) oil. (Note the advice on page 288 when using aromatherapy oils.)

Herbal remedies – Those that contain plant oestrogens or help to balance hormone levels are worth a try. They include black cohosh, motherwort, sage, wild yam, *Vitex agnus castus*, soy (as a concentrate made from beans or tofu), dong quai, nettle and red clover. Cypress tea (made by boiling crushed cypress cones in water for a few minutes) may make blood vessels less sensitive.

(Note the advice on page 277 when using herbal remedies.)

Tests and investigations

If necessary, your doctor will rule out other causes of flushing, such as a skin condition called rosacea, blushing due to embarrassment, oversensitivity to hot drinks or food, certain drugs, an overactive thyroid and two unusual disorders – carcinoid and phaeochromocytoma.

need to see a doctor?

See your doctor if flushes and sweats interfere with everyday activities or prevent you from sleeping properly.

Medical treatment

Taking HRT relieves flushes and sweats in nine in ten women but see page 36 for its side effects and page 303 for more detailed information about it.

your action plan

✔ **Vital**	✔ **Could be vital**	(✔) **Optional**
• Exercise	• Dietary changes	• Hydrotherapy
• Stress management	• Medical treatment	• Aromatherapy massage
• Exposure to light		• Herbal remedies

post-menopausal vaginal bleeding

Periods stop abruptly in some women but in many others they are spaced increasingly far apart until they eventually stop. You can't be sure (without hormone tests) that you've had your menopause until you've been period-free for a year. Post-menopausal bleeding can be an abnormally late period, but this is unlikely.

The biggest concern is whether bleeding is a sign of womb, cervix or ovary cancer. A woman who bleeds and is not on HRT has a 10 per cent risk of such a cancer, and a 10 per cent risk that something else important is wrong. Other possibilities include a womb or a cervix polyp or a fibroid (though fibroids generally shrink after the menopause). An inflamed cervix can be to blame, as can a sore vagina. A woman may not produce enough oestrogen to keep her vagina healthy, and eventually it can become inflamed

symptom sorter

Gynae or gynae-related causes of post-menopausal vaginal bleeding

● ● ● **Most likely** – HRT, the Pill, atrophic vulvo-vaginitis

● ● **Less likely** – womb surgery, some cervix treatments

● **Possible** – oestrogen-producing ovary cyst, womb or cervix polyp, cervix, womb or ovary cancer, stress

(see atrophic vulvo-vaginitis, page 174). She may also have itching and a watery, bloodstained discharge. Very occasionally, stress triggers bleeding and bleeding or a bloodstained discharge is common for a few weeks after womb surgery or some cervix treatments. Some women bleed if a hormone imbalance – such as from an oestrogen-producing ovarian cyst or wrongly prescribed oestrogen-only HRT – encourages the womb lining to thicken.

If you stay on the Pill in your late 40s or early 50s you are unlikely to confuse regular Pill-induced 'periods' with post-menopausal bleeding, as the latter tends to be irregular and unexpected but tell your doctor if you have any bleeding of this type.

When you start HRT, you may – depending on its type (see below) – expect 'periods'. But tell your doctor if in the first four to six months you also have spotting, though this is usually nothing to worry about.

If you start HRT while you are still having natural periods, your doctor will prescribe 'sequential combined' HRT. This provides daily oestrogen, with progestogen (which resembles progesterone) for 10-13 days every month or three months. You'll get a 'period' every month (or three months, depending on the formulation) when you finish the progestogen tablets or soon after. But tell your doctor if you have any change in your bleeding pattern or if you continue bleeding, as you may need investigations to discover why. If these reveal nothing your doctor may recommend a higher dose of progestogen to control the bleeding.

'Bleed-free' ('continuous combined') HRT is practical, and suitable if:

• you've been free from natural periods for a year

• you've taken sequential combined HRT for one or two years;

• your periods stopped before you went on sequential combined HRT

• you're over 54

It provides oestrogen and progestogen every day, so the womb lining never thickens enough to bleed. You may get a little bleeding at first, though this should stop after about six months. Tell your doctor if you start bleeding continuously, or if you bleed after being period-free.

what to do yourself

Help to keep hormone levels healthy by eating a healthy diet, maintaining a healthy weight, taking regular moderate exercise, managing stress wisely and going out in bright daylight.

Tests and investigations

Your doctor will examine you, take a cervical smear, and probably send you urgently to a gynaecologist for an ultrasound scan, and a hysteroscopy and womb-lining biopsy.

Medical treatment

This depends on the cause.

need to see a doctor?

Tell your doctor at once about any bleeding after you've been period-free for a year or about any irregular or otherwise unexpected bleeding if you are still on the Pill, or HRT.

your action plan

✔ **Vital**
• Medical assessment

✔ **Could be vital**
• Home and medical treatment

early menopause

An early menopause, meaning one that takes place between 40 and 45, is unusual but can be perfectly normal. However, a premature menopause (before 40) which happens to one woman in 100, usually indicates that something is wrong. A premature menopause is often called 'premature ovarian failure'. Unfortunately, both an early and a premature menopause can encourage osteoporosis, heart disease and strokes, so it's worth using lifestyle measures and, perhaps, medical therapy, to counteract these conditions.

Several things can provoke a premature or early menopause that's permanent:

• Single status – the average single woman has her menopause about two years earlier than the average partnered woman. This may be because single women are less likely to have had children, or to have been on the Pill for years. This means that over the years they have ovulated more, and therefore used up their eggs faster.

• Heavy smoking – this makes the menopause occur about two years earlier on average.

• Polycystic ovary syndrome (see page 139) – this encourages a relatively early menopause.

• Inflamed ovaries – this may happen with autoimmune disorders, such as an underactive thyroid (due to Hashimoto's thyroiditis, see page 252), Addison's disease (an adrenal gland disorder) and isolated autoimmune ovarian failure and with viral infection of the ovaries (such as with mumps).

• Sterilisation – this makes the menopause occur about two years earlier on average.

• Over-zealous removal of the womb lining during an operation called endometrial resection (or ablation).

• Hysterectomy – a woman who loses her womb but keeps her ovaries is likely to have her menopause up to five years early (two on average), possibly because it may interrupt the blood supply to her ovaries.

• Anti-cancer chemotherapy.

• Radiotherapy of an ovary – if done before the age of 30, for example, this makes the menopause occur an average of seven years earlier.

• Genetic mutations of certain types of ovary cell.

• Surgical removal of an ovary – if done before the age of 30, for example, this makes the menopause an average of seven years earlier.

For those circumstances in which periods never start, or which cause a reversible menopause, see 'Irregular, scanty or absent periods', page 108.

what to do yourself

Help prevent an early menopause by being a non-smoker and, if you have polycystic ovary syndrome or inflamed ovaries, arranging a suitable package of treatment. Do the same if your periods are becoming increasingly further apart, as this suggests that they might even stop altogether.

Tests and investigations

A premature menopause can be confirmed by at least two and preferably three sets of blood tests showing that your levels of gonadotrophins (follicle-stimulating hormone and luteinising hormone) are within the post-menopausal range. Sex chromosomes are investigated in a woman who has her menopause before 30. Any other tests and investigations needed depend on your symptoms and history.

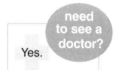 Yes. **need to see a doctor?**

Medical treatment

Your doctor may test your level of follicle-stimulating hormone to check that you are menopausal. The level is generally continuously high (at over 25 iu/l or more), indicating that your pituitary is trying desperately to make your 'failing' ovaries ovulate.

Treatment depends on what's made the menopause early but many women are advised to take HRT to reduce their raised risk of osteoporosis and, perhaps, heart disease. Modern fertility treatments enable some post-menopausal women to become pregnant.

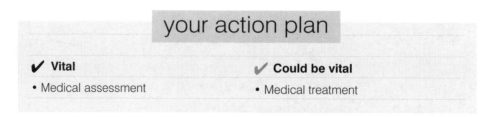

your action plan

✔ **Vital**
• Medical assessment

✔ **Could be vital**
• Medical treatment

non-gynae conditions with gynae side effects or links

The conditions discussed in this section either cause gynae symptoms, or result from changes in the reproductive system or sex-hormone levels. Some, including cystitis, leaking of urine, osteoporosis, eating disorders and irritable bowel syndrome, are covered in depth since they have such close gynae links. For others, including chronic fatigue syndrome, acne, and asthma we'll consider only their gynae links.

cystitis

The symptoms of cystitis arise from anything that irritates the lining of the bladder or urine passage (urethra) or makes the bladder muscle irritable. They include wanting to pass water frequently and urgently, even if there isn't much there. Passing urine causes a tingling sensation at first and a burning or stabbing pain later. If the bladder muscle is irritable the bladder tends to contract intermittently, so you may have to urinate urgently and may leak if you can't get to the toilet in time. You may have low stomach-ache, backache and a fever and feel generally unwell. Severe inflammation of the bladder's lining may make the urine bloodstained and infected urine may be cloudy, bloodstained or smelly.

Most likely causes

A urine infection – this means bacteria are clinging to the bladder lining, multiplying there and making it inflamed. Usually they come from the vulva (though they originate from the bowel) and the culprit is *E. coli* (*Escherichia coli*). Urine infection is common – indeed nearly six in 10 American women, for example, have one at some time. *However, only one woman in two with cystitis has an infection.* Also, while one in 20 young sexually active women has *E. coli* in her urine, in most these bacteria are transitory and only 8 per cent of these women get cystitis. A sexually transmitted infection such as chlamydia can irritate the bladder and/or urethra.

Vigorous thrusting of the penis may irritate the urethra and bladder neck (which are close to the vagina's front wall) and push bacteria from the vulva up the urethra to the bladder. Cystitis is most common after the first experience of sex (when it's called 'honeymoon cystitis') and sex with a new partner. The more partners you have, the more likely repeated cystitis is.

Alcohol and **methylxanthines** (including caffeine) in tea, coffee and cola can trigger a strong urge to urinate.

Stress raises your adrenaline level, which stimulates the bladder.

Feeling cold makes many of us urinate more often, partly because we don't sweat as much and partly because it's a stress trigger.

Less likely causes

Irritation of the urethra – possibly by toiletries, spermicide, traces of washing powder and swimming-pool chlorine.

Pressure on the bladder – This could be a diaphragm, tampon, pregnancy (cystitis usually lessens after three months), fibroid, or prolapse perhaps preventing the bladder from emptying properly and so encouraging bacteria to breed.

A low or falling oestrogen level – this can make the lining of the urethra thinner and drier, which makes the bladder neck and urethra more readily irritated by sex or other causes and explains why cystitis is especially likely on certain types of Pill and after the menopause (see urethral syndrome, page 174). It can also cause dryness and inflammation around the urethral opening, which encourages the colonisation of the vagina with mainly *E. coli* instead of mainly lactobacilli, and encourages urine infection.

Diabetes – if this is either unrecognised or poorly treated, it causes high sugar levels in urine, which increase urine volume and irritate the bladder. Possible signs include abnormal thirst or fatigue, frequent passing of urine, itching, numbness or pins and needles in hands and feet, and deteriorating eyesight.

Interstitial cystitis (IC) – this affects nine times as many women as men and is a long-term inflammation of the bladder wall. It causes more or less continuous cystitis, perhaps with extreme urgency, frequency, painful urination and sex and pain in the abdominal, urethral or vaginal areas. At worst, the bladder lining ulcerates. The cause is unclear. One suggestion is that the bladder lining's protective layer of mucus isn't thick enough, encouraging little tears in the bladder lining which allow irritating substances to enter the bladder wall. Another is that IC is an autoimmune disorder. The first attack often begins after a urine infection that doesn't respond to antibiotics. It tends to go spontaneously in around one in two women.

Other causes

● **Certain foods or drinks** – Irritation of the bladder and urethra can be caused by tomatoes, most fruits (not melon or pears), dairy food, spices, chocolate, artificial sweeteners, herbal teas, vinegar and certain food additives and seasonings.

● Smoking

● Urine stones

● A catheter (urine drain)

● Bladder tumour

● Endometriosis

● Pelvic inflammatory disease

● Ovary cyst, fibroids, prolapse

● Ovary, womb or vulva cancer

● **Threadworms** – most likely in young girls

● **Flukes** – these are parasitic worms, contracted when paddling or swimming in certain lakes or rivers in Africa, Asia, Spain, Portugal or Greece.

symptom sorter

Gynae or gynae-related causes of cystitis

●●● **Most likely** – urine infection, bruised bladder or urethra from vigorous thrusting of the penis, alcohol, tea, coffee, cola, stress, feeling cold

●● **Less likely** – irritation of urethra by toiletries, spermicide, traces of washing powder, or swimming-pool chlorine, pressure from a diaphragm, tampon, pregnancy, fibroid, or prolapse, dry vagina and vulva, low or falling oestrogen level on certain types of Pill or after menopause, urethral syndrome, diabetes, interstitial cystitis

● **Possible** – certain foods, urine stones, a catheter, bladder tumour, endometriosis, ovary cyst, fibroids, prolapse, ovary or womb cancer, threadworms, flukes

what to do yourself

Identify and avoid the trigger and treat the cause, if possible. The following tips should help prevent and/or treat cystitis:

Adjust fluid intake – Each day drink at least 1.5 litres (just over 2 ½ pints) and preferably 2-3 litres (3 ½ – 5 ¼ pints) a day of fluid (not counting milk or alcohol) – more if the weather is hot and dry or you exercise a lot. Your urine will be copious and pale if you are well hydrated. A good fluid intake helps to prevent a high concentration of any irritating substances in the urine. Reducing your intake of coffee, tea, cola and alcohol (or choosing decaffeinated coffee) may also help to prevent cystitis.

During an attack – Drink even more to help flush out infecting bacteria or other irritating substances. Start with around 0.5 litre (about a pint) of water, then have a glass every 20 minutes for three hours. Lemon barley water is a good alternative: make this by boiling 100g (4oz) of pot barley in water for 45 minutes, then straining, cooling and adding the juice and finely grated peel of two lemons and a little honey to taste. Don't be concerned that these acidic fruits will irritate your bladder, since acidic foods do not make the urine more acidic.

Make your urine less acid to help prevent stinging, by putting a teaspoon of sodium bicarbonate (baking soda) in every third glass of fluid or taking potassium citrate mixture or a flavoured cystitis remedy containing potassium citrate (from a pharmacy).

Dietary changes – Eat plenty of foods rich in antioxidants (see page 259). Also, eat more foods rich in omega-3 fatty acids (see page 256) and less food rich in omega-6s, but reduce your overall intake of fat, especially the saturated variety. If you suspect a particular food, avoid it for two weeks to see if this helps, taking care that your diet remains nutritious. All this helps to counter any infection and/or inflammation.

During an attack, avoid sugary, spicy and acidic foods.

For recurrent urine infections, drink a daily half-glass of cranberry juice or take cranberry-extract tablets (they should be free from added sugar, and are available from pharmacies and health stores). The cranberry's proanthocyanidin pigments help to prevent bacteria from sticking to the bladder lining. Also, eat asparagus, beetroot and raw garlic to counteract infection.

Stop smoking – to see whether this discourages cystitis, since it has been suggested that chemicals in urine that are derived from inhaled smoke may irritate the bladder.

Sex tips – Wash your vulva and around your anus before sex and ask your partner to wash his penis. Empty your bladder before and within half an hour after sex. Drink a glass of water before and after sex to help flush out any bacteria that may enter the bladder during sex. Before penetration, ensure you are aroused and that your vulva and vagina are well lubricated. Try different positions for intercourse.

Clothing tips – Wear cotton knickers and loose trousers and avoid tights or wear ones with a cotton gusset. Avoid any clothes that press on your waist or tummy or the opening of your urethra.

Empty your bladder completely – when you urinate and always urinate sitting, as it's harder to empty your bladder properly when 'hovering' above a toilet seat to avoid touching it with your bottom. Urinate every two hours during the day and before you go to bed at night.

Wipe your bottom from front to back – to help to prevent urine infection.

Wash after opening your bowels – when possible, or use a moist cleansing wipe.

Take showers – rather than bathing if possible.

Manage stress – If stress exacerbates your symptoms, empty your bladder before stressful situations and aim to manage stress more effectively.

Heat and cold – During an attack, keep warm and ease any stomach ache with a covered hot-water bottle or electrically heated pad. Some people find that a cold compress (a flannel soaked in cold water and frequently refreshed) over their lower abdomen is more soothing.

Avoid certain toiletries – If toiletries or washing powder are to blame, try using use unperfumed soap, avoid 'feminine-hygiene' toiletries and bubble bath, choose white toilet paper (coloured paper contains dyes that might irritate) and rinse clothes well when laundering.

Exercise – Take a daily half hour's exercise to improve your circulation – and therefore your health, including that of your bladder (see page 263).

Take painkillers – if necessary.

Hydrotherapy – Boost your pelvic circulation with regular contrast sitz baths (see page 275). This may help prevent and treat cystitis.

Massage and aromatherapy – Ease tension and pain by massaging your abdomen with two drops each of juniper and lavender oils in two teaspoons of warmed sweet almond or other carrier oil. (Note the advice on page 288 when using aromatherapy oils.)

Herbal remedies – At the first sign of infection, drink a cup of *uva ursi* or juniper berry tea three times a day. If using *uva ursi* take cranberry juice or extract too, as this helps *uva ursi* to work better. Horsetail is a good alternative if you don't have an infection. (Note the advice on page 277 when using herbal remedies.)

Pain relief and relaxation – In addition to the above measures, take over-the-counter painkillers if necessary. Also, try to distract your mind with interesting activities. Use relaxation techniques so that muscle tension does not worsen your pain.

Tests and investigations

A 'dipstick' test in the doctor's surgery isn't reliable enough but a laboratory urine test will show whether you have an infection (and which antibiotics are likely to work).

For recurrent infections it's wise to have your urine tested again 7-10 days after a course of antibiotics and to have a urine-sugar test to rule out diabetes. If necessary, your doctor will rule out other possibilities, then arrange a cystoscopy (examination of the bladder through a viewing tube passed up the urethra). This is the only way of diagnosing IC.

> **need to see a doctor?**
>
> See your doctor if home treatment makes you no better within 48 hours, if you have a temperature, severe pain, kidney disease, or repeated attacks or if you pass blood.

Medical treatment

Suspected infections are treated with a short course of suitable antibiotics, started at once and changed if they don't help or, perhaps, if test results favour an alternative antibiotic.

Other treatments depend on the cause.

There is no cure for IC, but several treatments may help. Oral medication with prescription-strength non-steroidal anti-inflammatory drugs, antispasmodic, muscle-relaxant, or antihistamine drugs, or pentosan polysulfate sodium (available in the USA), may help. Dimethyl sulfoxide (DMSO, an anti-inflammatory) or sodium hyaluronate (which counteracts any deficiency of the mucus lining the bladder) can be squirted into the bladder through a cystoscope. Certain antidepressants can help to relieve pain. Cimetidine (a stomach-ulcer drug) may be useful. Surgical techniques include distending the urethra and bladder under general anaesthesia.

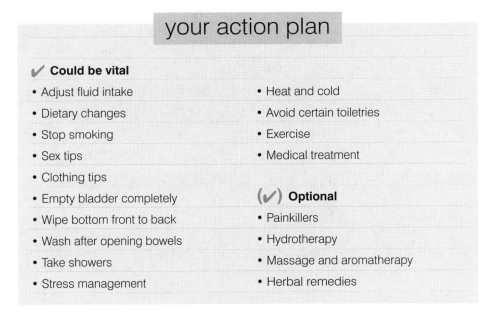

your action plan

✔ Could be vital

- Adjust fluid intake
- Dietary changes
- Stop smoking
- Sex tips
- Clothing tips
- Empty bladder completely
- Wipe bottom front to back
- Wash after opening bowels
- Take showers
- Stress management

- Heat and cold
- Avoid certain toiletries
- Exercise
- Medical treatment

(✔) Optional

- Painkillers
- Hydrotherapy
- Massage and aromatherapy
- Herbal remedies

leaking (incontinence)

This is an annoying, frustrating and embarrassing problem but one that is relatively common. One in two women who leak has stress incontinence, one in three has urge incontinence and the rest have both. The good news is that up to three in four women can become dry or drier.

Stress incontinence

This is due to weakness of the muscle around the top of the urethra that keeps urine in the bladder and of the pelvic floor muscles which support the bladder neck and urethra. Activities such as sneezing, coughing, laughing, lifting, rising from a chair, jumping, starting sex or straining when opening your bowels raise the pressure in the abdomen and therefore on the bladder. A difficult delivery, several close pregnancies, or a hysterectomy can weaken the pelvic floor, as can being overweight, a poor diet, repeated coughing, ageing, a low post-menopausal oestrogen level and severe constipation. Some women also have frequency and urgency – meaning that they need to pass urine more frequently and/or urgently than normal – as well as leaking.

Urge incontinence ('detrusor instability')

This means that the bladder-wall muscle is overactive or irritable and may sometimes empty suddenly, completely and uncontrollably. Frequency and urgency are other possibilities, as is wetting the bed at night and finding you can't get to the lavatory in time during the day, which is most likely with a urine infection. Other triggers include stress, smoking, orgasm, diabetes, certain foods and drinks (strong tea or coffee, cola, alcohol, fruit juice, spicy foods, sugar and dairy products), certain drugs (including diuretics – 'water tablets') and pelvic surgery. Unreliability may also be due to a low oestrogen level or a problem with the bladder's nerves.

what to do yourself

Exercise – Take a half hour's exercise daily to improve your circulation and therefore your general health, including that of your pelvic floor and bladder.

Buy highly absorbent pads to cope with leaks.

Dietary changes – Eat foods rich in plant oestrogens to boost low oestrogen levels after the menopause, and eat more foods rich in antioxidants and omega-3 fatty acids and less food rich in omega-6s, to reduce any inflammation.

Avoid eating or drinking anything which you think might irritate your bladder.

Healthy weight maintenance – Lose any excess weight as stress incontinence is more common in overweight women.

No smoking – Stop smoking, since repeated coughing due to irritation of the airways encourages stress incontinence.

Pelvic-floor exercises – If you have stress incontinence, do several sets of pelvic floor exercises five times a day (see page 265).

symptom sorter

Gynae or gynae-related causes of leaking urine

- ● ● ● **Most likely** – weak muscles around bladder neck, urine infection, stress, smoking, orgasm (fluid may actually be sexual ejaculation, not urine), diabetes, certain foods and drinks, overactive bladder
- ● ● **Less likely** – low oestrogen level (urethral syndrome), certain drugs
- ● **Possible** – overactive thyroid, after pelvic surgery, bladder-nerve disorder

Vaginal cones – Consider strengthening your pelvic-floor muscles further by learning to hold in your vagina, for 30 minutes at a time, a 'vaginal cone' from a set of cones of different weights (see the Helplist on page 315).

Bladder training – Holding in urine for progressively longer intervals can help urge incontinence. Start by going once an hour, then lengthen the interval day by day until you can hold on for three or four hours.

Exposure to light – Get some bright outdoor daylight each day to encourage a healthy hormone balance.

Hydrotherapy, heat and cold – Have regular contrast sitz baths (see page 275) to boost your pelvic circulation and muscle tone.

Try using a 'Contiform' (see Helplist, page 314) – This plastic tampon-like device can help to prevent leaks and at the same time promote pelvic-floor fitness.

Tests and investigations

These may include urine and blood tests, vaginal and rectal examinations and measurements of bladder capacity and urine flow.

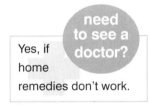

need to see a doctor?

Yes, if home remedies don't work.

Medical treatment

Stress incontinence. Possibilities include electro-stimulation of the nerves to the pelvic floor or bladder from a device inserted in your vagina, a ring-shaped oestrogen-releasing vaginal pessary, or taking HRT or wearing a U-shaped pessary to hold your bladder neck in place.

There are several surgical options. One is an operation (colposuspension) to secure a sagging vagina that's causing leaking by pulling on the bladder neck. Another, the tension-free vaginal tape (TVT) procedure, for persistent stress incontinence, introduces a sling of tape – through two small cuts in the abdomen and one in the vagina's front wall – to support the urethra; the tape is then threaded around the urethra and fixed to provide support. The TVT operation seems to be successful in over four in five women and the cure rates at six months for colposuspension and TVT are about the same. However, one study suggests that postoperative complications are more likely and recovery takes longer after colposuspension and bladder injury is more common during TVT.

You could have injections of collagen or fat around your bladder neck. However, one study found that only 28 per cent of women who had these were dry a year afterwards, 16 per cent leaked only once a month, and two in three improved a little.

Urge incontinence. Your doctor may recommend a drug such as tolterodine to calm your bladder or electrical stimulation of the nerves to your pelvic floor or bladder from a device in your vagina.

your action plan

✔ **Vital**	• Healthy weight	• Exposure to light
• Exercise	maintenance	• Medical treatment
	• No smoking	
✔ **Could be vital**	• Pelvic-floor exercises	(✔) **Optional**
• Highly absorbent pads	• Vaginal cones	• Hydrotherapy, heat,
• Dietary changes	• Bladder training	and cold

osteoporosis

Osteoporosis is a condition in which the bones gradually lose minerals, making them light and fragile. Bones affected by osteoporosis fracture readily and one in three women over 50 will have an osteoporotic fracture, compared with only one man in 12. Osteoporosis also encourages the spine to bend and crumble, leading to pain, a 'dowager's hump' and loss of height.

Bone mineral-density normally peaks when a woman is in her late 20s, starts falling in her 30s, and drops faster after the menopause as sex hormone levels fall.

Risk factors for osteoporosis include:

* age

* a premature or early menopause

* a long time without periods – for example, with anorexia or too much exercise. (pregnancy and breastfeeding don't count)

* smoking – partly because it advances the menopause by an average of two years

* too little exercise – since bone-strength depends on the stimulation of the pull from muscles

* prolonged rest – for the same reason

* too little outdoor light – as for people who are housebound and those who are dark-skinned or wear all-enveloping clothes, live in very northerly or southerly latitudes or don't get enough vitamin D in their diet

* a poor diet – as this doesn't include enough bone-friendly nutrients

* repeated, poor-quality slimming diets

* too much alcohol on a regular basis

* a small thin frame

* anorexia

* osteoporosis in the family

* long-term high-dose steroids (for example, for severe asthma)

* cancer, a liver or thyroid disorder, rheumatoid arthritis or any gut disorder which prevents nutrients from being properly absorbed

* certain drugs (for example, for schizophrenia)

what to do yourself

Simple lifestyle measures can strengthen bones or prevent further weakening.

Dietary changes – Eat plenty of foods rich in bone-friendly nutrients – calcium, magnesium, zinc, vitamins C, D (oily fish, egg yolk, full-fat dairy foods, nuts, cold-pressed vegetable oils, fortified food – such as breakfast cereal, and margarine) and K (liver, eggs, green leafy vegetables, cauliflower, turnips, beans, whole grains), and plant pigments. Bone density is lost around the menopause much more slowly in women with a high intake of plant oestrogens (see page 260). Avoid added salt and sugar, coffee, fizzy drinks, alcohol, red meat, processed meats and refined carbohydrate.

Healthy weight maintenance – Ideally, always eat a sensible diet and if you go on a slimming diet, make sure it's nutritious.

No smoking – This is vital for healthy bones.

Exercise – Take regular weight-bearing exercise (such as skipping, dancing or tennis) to raise the bone mineral density in your legs, hips and spine.

Strength training is vital for older people as it makes muscles more powerful and strengthens bones. Examples include sitting down and bending your knees as you lift a weight with your feet, or lying on one side and raising your upper leg with a weight strapped to its ankle. Do three sets of eight repetitions of each movement. This is best done three times a week.

Exposure to light – Get some bright natural daylight on your bare skin each day to boost vitamin D production and so aid your bones' calcium uptake.

Food supplements – If you have a high risk of osteoporosis, or have the disease, consider taking a multivitamin and mineral product that includes vitamins D and K, calcium, magnesium, boron, silica and zinc.

Tests and investigations

X-rays can detect fractures. A bone-density scan (a DEXA or dual energy X-ray absorptiometry scan, which uses X-rays of two different powers) is the most reliable way of assessing bone strength and fracture risk. A urine test can show if bone is breaking down too fast.

need to see a doctor?

Yes, if you suspect osteoporosis because early recognition and treatment makes it less likely to progress and cause pain, fractures and deformity.

Medical treatment

If after the menopause you have osteoporosis, or have a risk of getting it, your doctor may recommend HRT. However, HRT increases the risk of womb cancer and, perhaps, breast cancer. Also, a recent overview of many studies suggests that if HRT is to prevent fractures, you have to start it soon after the menopause, and continue for the rest of your life.

Alternatives to HRT include:

• bisphosphonates such as alendronate and etidronate, which help to prevent the action of bone-destroying cells and are possibly the most effective drugs

• SERMs (selective oestrogen re-uptake modulators) such as raloxifene, which reduces the risk of osteoporosis causing fractures of the spine, without encouraging breast cancer. (Note, though, that while raloxifene, for example, can increase bone mineral density, reduce a high cholesterol level and decrease the risk of breast and womb cancer, it can trigger hot flushes, and – like HRT – raises the risk of abnormal blood clots.)

• tibolone – a synthetic steroid that helps to prevent osteoporosis, and also helps to prevent menopausal hot flushes and night sweats

• vitamin D and calcium supplements.

your action plan

✔ Vital

• Dietary changes
• Healthy weight
  maintenance
• No smoking

• Exercise
• Exposure to light

✔ Could be vital

• Medical treatment

(✔) Optional

• Food supplements

anaemia

Iron-deficiency anaemia is the most common type, partly because one in 25 women is short of iron. Mild anaemia causes few, if any, problems, so is often unrecognised until a routine blood test. Severe anaemia can, however, make you tired, pale and even breathless on exertion. You may also have a sore tongue and soreness of the corners of the mouth, your nails may be thin and brittle, without their normal side-to-side convexity and your periods may be heavy.

Common causes of anaemia include a lack of iron-rich foods and heavy periods. Anaemia's link with periods can be a vicious circle for, while anaemia causes heavy periods that, in turn, worsen anaemia, heavy periods also cause anaemia that, in turn, worsens heavy periods. Other possible causes include bleeding – such as from continued slight blood loss from the gut (perhaps associated with gluten sensitivity, see page 250), poor absorption of iron from the gut and any serious illness. Stress can cause both poor digestion and poor absorption of iron and advanced gynae cancers can also cause anaemia.

what to do yourself

Dietary changes – Eat more foods rich in iron and, to aid its absorption, vitamin C, and copper (beans, peas, green vegetables, avocados, liver, shellfish, cheese, egg yolk, wholegrains, apricots, cherries, figs, nuts and olives). Cooking in stainless steel or non-enamel-coated cast-iron pans may raise your iron intake.

Only drink coffee, tea, cola, and alcohol (if at all) between meals, as they can reduce iron absorption.

Treat periods, if heavy – to avoid the vicious circle of anaemia-heavy periods-anaemia.

Stress management – Use effective strategies to make mealtimes more relaxed occasions.

Tests and investigations

You need blood tests to measure your iron levels.

> **need to see a doctor?**
> Yes, if you feel unwell and, perhaps, suspect anaemia.

Medical treatment

You may need iron medication for three to six months to replenish your iron stores.

your action plan

✔ Vital
- Treat periods, if heavy
- Stress management

✔ Could be vital
- Dietary changes
- Medical treatment

overweight and obesity

More than two in three women in the UK are overweight or obese and the picture is the same in many other westernised countries and worse in the USA.

But what's wrong with being fat and happy? For one thing, the two have no connection – overweight people are just as likely as anyone else to feel sad, angry or desperate and some 'comfort eat' to bury challenging emotions. Also, being overweight can be uncomfortable, tiring, and hard on feet and joints and health problems are very slightly more likely if your body mass index (BMI, see page 241) is 25-30, more likely if it's 30-35, and very much more likely if it's over 35.

Some of the health problems that could stem from being overweight include certain gynae conditions, such as heavy, irregular or painful periods, lumpy breasts, polycystic ovary syndrome, fertility problems, fibroids, and breast and womb cancers. They also include many 'non-gynae' conditions, such as indigestion, backache, snoring, varicose veins, diabetes, osteoarthritis, high blood pressure, asthma, heart disease, strokes and some cancers.

what to do yourself

Take in less energy from food than your body uses. You could do this just by eating fewer calories but it's much easier to lose weight and keep it off if you exercise each day, and learn how to deal with the triggers that make you overeat or eat too much comfort food.

Focus on keeping off lost pounds – Losing weight isn't usually too difficult – the challenge is keeping it off, since 95 per cent of successful slimmers regain their lost weight within a year. Many women who do this time and again testify to the discipline and self-denial of each new diet and the subsequent disappointment or despair as the pounds pile back on.

If you aim to make healthy eating and exercising habits permanent fixtures and not just something you occasionally do to get slim again, you will join the elite 5 per cent that remain slim. Of course you'll put on a few pounds now and then, but when you do, use the permanently slim person's secrets (see overleaf).

the permanently slim person's two secrets

1. When you overeat or put on two or three pounds, don't waste time feeling guilty and downhearted and then let your mood sabotage your diet by triggering comfort eating. Return immediately to a healthy weight-management programme.

2. Discover what food intake and balance, meal patterns, amount of rest and exercise, stress-management strategies and motivation and support are most helpful to healthy-weight maintenance for you as an individual.

Drink plenty – Even slight dehydration makes you burn fewer calories, so drink enough to keep your urine very pale.

Exercise – Move about more and take half an hour a day, at least five times a week, of aerobic activity. This burns calories immediately, raises your metabolic rate for hours and helps you to feel better and less prone to comfort eat. Choose 'low-impact' exercise (walking rather than jogging, for example) to protect your already burdened joints.

Regular muscle-strengthening exercise is vital too, as it builds extra muscle and muscle burns more energy than other tissue.

Exercise gives you a natural high and stops you craving food when you are not really hungry. Tests show that an obese woman's brain cells contain relatively few receptors for dopamine – a neurotransmitter that helps to regulate hunger. They also show that the fatter a woman is, the fewer of these receptors she has. When dopamine receptors are in short supply, dopamine can't work. But scientists believe exercise increases the number of receptors, so increasing dopamine activity and, perhaps, reducing the desire to overeat.

Stress management – Aim to recognise the emotions and situations that trigger comfort eating and work out a choice of effective strategies for dealing with them. Think of yourself as someone precious who deserves time spent on her. If comfort eating is a problem, keep handy a list of other things to do when the urge arises.

Aim for a sensible rate of weight loss – After the first week of a diet, when weight loss may be high because of fluid loss, aim to lose an average of 1–2 pounds (0.5–1kg) a week. Some weeks you may lose less, especially if you tend to gain weight before a period (perhaps because you eat more refined carbohydrate, eat more than usual, or retain fluid then). In other weeks – for example, after your period starts – you may lose more. However, if you regularly lose more, you may be losing muscle as well as fat and, perhaps, fluid, and that isn't good for your muscle strength, metabolic rate, bone strength, or body shape.

Keep your waist trim – 'Apple-shaped' women with a plump waist are more likely to develop polycystic ovaries and heart disease than are 'pear-shaped' ones with plump hips and thighs but a slim waist. Over-40s should aim to keep their waist less than 80cm (31½ in) and not over 88cm (34½ in).

Exposure to light – For comfort eating, go out in bright light each day to boost 'feel-good' endorphins and help balance neurotransmitters such as serotonin. Also, consider wearing a special mask programmed to flash red lights, for up to 30 minutes a day (see also page 291 and Helplist, page 315); this can aid relaxation, and aid weight loss.

For winter depression – (at worst, seasonal affective disorder, or SAD), if this makes you crave sweet, starchy foods (perhaps especially in the late afternoon and evening) or 'comfort eat' (eat because this makes you feel less low), get more bright outdoor daylight – preferably sunlight – to help balance neurotransmitters and hormones. Also, consider using a light visor or box.

For any obesity – get more bright outdoor daylight, as UV stimulates the thyroid, which helps to burn calories by raising the body's metabolic rate.

Dietary changes – If your physical activity level stays the same, you need to eat fewer calories but eat regularly, so that you don't get so hungry that you stuff yourself with easy-to-prepare sweet, fatty or starchy foods.

Eat a healthy diet with more low-calorie food, for example more vegetables and fruits and less fat, and replace red meat with poultry, fish and game. This way your plate will be fuller than before. (Don't eat too little fat, though, as this could encourage depression and hormone imbalance; 30 per cent of your daily calories should come from fats – see also page 255 – and it's vital to eat some foods rich in omega-3 fatty acids each day).

Favour foods with a low glycaemic index (GI, see page 261). If you eat high-GI food, have only small amounts, and eat some low-GI food as well. This will help you feel fuller for longer, smooth out blood sugar swings, foster healthy levels of insulin,

symptom sorter

Gynae or gynae-related causes of overweight and obesity

● ● ● **Most likely** – fluid retention, premenstrual syndrome, pregnancy, polycystic ovary syndrome

● ● **Less likely** – oestrogen dominance (cyclical gain), oestrogen deficiency (non-cyclical gain)

● **Possible** – ovary cyst, fibroids, underactive thyroid

and reduce your risk of polycystic ovary syndrome and diabetes. It's natural to like sweet, satisfying, 'feel-good' food and 'comfort' foods made with white flour but overindulgence is fattening. So have items such as cakes, biscuits, pastry, puddings and ice cream at the end of a nutritious meal containing low-GI foods that you've eaten slowly, so that you feel relatively full. In one study, researchers found that the most effective meal for staving off hunger was a vegetable omelette followed by fruit, and the food most likely to make you hungry quickly was instant porridge!

Choose highly nutritious foods over those with lots of calories from refined carbohydrates and animal fats but few other nutrients since, with your increased bulk, you need more nutrients to keep you healthy than does someone your height with a healthy weight. Also, because you have a lot of body fat, you need plenty of foods rich in antioxidants to prevent free radicals from damaging your fat. As you lose weight continue to eat plenty of foods rich in antioxidants to counteract the free-radical-raising effects of toxins released from stored fat.

Be cautious over low-fat weight-loss diets. One study showed that women on a 1,200 calories-a-day, moderate-fat diet (meaning 35 per cent of daily calories from fats) were much more successful in keeping off their lost weight than those on a 1,200 calorie-a-day, *low-fat* diet (with only 20 per cent of calories from fats). This is probably because fat improves mood and make us feel fuller faster and for longer.

Get a slimming buddy or join a slimming club – Some women benefit from the support of a friend with the same goal. Many more find a slimming club's tips, encouragement and support a great help, although most women stop going when they've lost weight then start putting it back on, whereas it's better to keep going or to return when you've gained only a few pounds.

Know your body mass index (BMI) – To work this out (adults only) note your weight in kilograms then multiply your height in metres by itself and divide your weight by this number. (For pounds and inches, multiply your weight in pounds by 703, then divide this by your height in inches squared – which means multiplied by itself).

If your BMI is 20-25, your weight is healthy. If it's 25-30, you are overweight. If it's over 30, you're obese. Some people are naturally plump but the range of weights that constitute a healthy BMI of 20-25 allows for differences in build.

Food supplements – Consider taking a daily multivitamin and mineral supplement, as your increased bulk may mean you need more of these nutrients than your diet provides.

Massage and aromatherapy – Each day, either do three minutes of dry skin brushing over any dimpled fat ('cellulite') on hips, thighs and upper arms, to boost the local circulation. Or massage these areas with firm strokes plus light pats, lubricating with three drops of geranium, fennel, rosemary, juniper, grapefruit or lime oil added to two teaspoons of sweet almond or other carrier oil. (Note the advice on page 288 when using aromatherapy oils.)

Hydrotherapy, heat and cold – Use a loofah or body-brush over cellulite in the bath. Or boost your circulation by having a shower that's alternately comfortably hot (for a minute or two) then cool (for 10 seconds or so).

Tests and investigations

Regular weight checks may help. You may need a blood test to check your thyroid hormones. Other possibilities depend on whether any other problems are suspected.

need to see a doctor? Yes, if you remain fat or repeatedly put on a lot of weight and lose it again.

Medical treatment

Your doctor can help you to find effective weight-loss and healthy-weight maintenance programmes. These could include help with stress-management strategies from a counsellor. Diet drugs such as orlistat and silbutramine are suitable for some obese people. As a last resort, some very obese people have their stomach made smaller or have fat in certain areas surgically removed.

your action plan

✔ **Vital**	✔ **Could be vital**	(✔) **Optional**
• Focus on keeping off lost pounds	• Dietary changes	• Know your BMI
• Drink plenty	• A slimming buddy or club	• Food supplements
• Exercise	• Medical treatment	• Massage and aromatherapy
• Stress management		• Hydrotherapy, heat and cold
• Aim for a sensible rate of weight loss		
• Keep your waist trim		
• Light		

binge-eating, compulsive overeating and bulimia

Regular bingeing can lead to overweight or obesity and, perhaps, gynae conditions such as heavy, irregular, painful or absent periods, lumpy breasts, polycystic ovary syndrome, fertility problems, fibroids and breast and womb cancers. It may also be associated with bulimia.

Bulimia ('the appetite of an ox') involves two factors. One is repeated bingeing, almost always on carbohydrates and fats. The other is vomiting or taking laxatives to get rid of the food. One in 100 girls develops bulimia at some time, usually in her late teens or early 20s.

The usual trigger is stress in the family or at school. Other people may not realise that you are facing a challenge. You long to improve matters and cope with your sadness, loneliness, anger, fear or perceived inadequacy or imperfection. Yet you feel powerless, so instead you may eat compulsively, or diet. This fans physical hunger for sweet, starchy, fatty food. So you binge. This makes you feel even more out of control. Now you try to take control (and, perhaps, punish yourself for 'failing') by vomiting or taking laxatives.

All this disrupts body chemistry, making it hard to recognise feelings of hunger and fullness. You may develop stomach pain, corroded teeth, frequent throat infections, bloating and fatigue as well as any of the gynae conditions mentioned above.

Many women with bulimia have symptoms like those of SAD (seasonal affective disorder or winter depression – in which a lack of bright light disrupts neurotransmitters such as serotonin). It's interesting that the foods binged on by people with bulimia are the very ones craved by those with SAD. Perhaps, as with SAD, the disrupted body chemistry associated with bulimia may improve if you get more bright daylight; certainly light therapy can greatly reduce the frequency of bingeing.

what to do yourself

Dietary changes – Eat regular, healthy, appetising, attractive meals, with plenty of foods rich in calcium, magnesium, zinc, vitamins B and C. Eat more foods rich in omega-3 fatty acids (see page 256) and less foods rich in omega-6s; this enables normal serotonin production. Most importantly, favour foods with a low glycaemic-index (GI – see page 261) and if you must eat high-GI foods, have only small amounts and some low-GI food too. This will help you to feel fuller for longer, smooth out blood-sugar swings and reduce your risk of polycystic ovary syndrome and diabetes.

If you want to lose weight, look after yourself by eating a very nutritious diet, and note that exercise may be particularly helpful.

Exercise – Take daily aerobic exercise to give yourself a natural 'high' and curb your appetite.

Stress management – Try to establish, with the help of a trusted relative, friend, doctor or counsellor if necessary, a choice of ways of managing stress more effectively and in non-damaging ways. Ideas include learning to recognise and accept your feelings and, perhaps, to direct them into more positive outlets; keeping a diary to pinpoint binge triggers and coming up with activities you can easily do instead of bingeing.

Exposure to bright light – Go outside in bright light for longer each day, and consider using a light visor or box.

Tests and investigations

If any are necessary, the choice depends on what, if any, are your symptoms. For bulimia, for example, you may need tests for the levels of certain nutrients.

need to see a doctor?

Yes, if you are unhappy or unwell.

Medical treatment

Your doctor may recommend that you see a therapist for a type of psychological counselling called cognitive-behavioural therapy. This would aim to help you view your situation and your solution to it in a different light, so giving you a different perspective on your circumstances and helping you find alternatives to compulsive overeating or bingeing as ways of managing stress. Combining this with taking an SSRI (selective serotonin reuptake inhibitor) antidepressant – which increases the availability of serotonin in the body – could be even more helpful.

your action plan

✔ **Vital**

• Dietary changes

• Exercise

• Stress management

• Exposure to bright light

✔ **Could be vital**

• Medical treatment

anorexia

Around one in 100 teenagers, mostly girls, suffer from anorexia at some time. They become extremely underweight by drastically reducing their food intake in spite of hunger. Once a girl's weight falls below a certain level her periods stop, and she may feel cold and develop a hairy back.

Many people see stopping eating as the only way they can manage stress. At that time in their life they are simply unable to access non-damaging ways of dealing with themselves and their situation. Limiting food intake helps them to suppress emotional pain and feel more in control but it isn't a good solution. It endangers their health and, at worst, it can kill.

what to do yourself

You need nutritious and attractive meals rich in zinc (as your levels of this may be low); bright daylight and gentle daily exercise may be beneficial. You also need help to understand what's happening, put your life into perspective and work out a choice of non-damaging yet effective ways of facing life's challenges other than by curbing food intake.

Tests and investigations

The doctor will rule out other causes of weight loss and arrange specialised help, perhaps at an eating disorders unit.

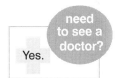

Yes.

need to see a doctor?

Medical treatment

Your doctor's most important job is to ensure that you do not die from starvation, so they will recommend frequent high-calorie meals, with supervision to make sure that you eat them. When your weight is healthy again, you may benefit from anti-depressant drugs and psychological therapy. Treatment generally includes one-to-one or group counselling or psychotherapy, plus family counselling or therapy.

your action plan

✔ **Vital**

• Medical treatment

• Nutritious, attractive meals

✔ **Could be vital**

• Gentle daily exercise

• Exposure to light

• Counselling or psychotherapy

irritable bowel syndrome

One person in three occasionally has an 'irritable' bowel, and one in five people with an irritable bowel has such frequent trouble that they are said to have irritable bowel syndrome (IBS). This means some combination of:

• stomach-ache (usually eased by emptying bowels or passing wind)

• mucus in bowel motions

- constipation, diarrhoea (especially early in the morning) or alternating diarrhoea and constipation

- a sensation that the bowels are never empty

- wind and bloating for hours after eating

Diarrhoea, constipation and pain partly result from poor co-ordination of bowel-wall muscle contractions that prevents the smooth passage of food. Pain also results from unusual sensitivity of bowel nerves to stretching. The bowel is unusually sensitive to triggers such as changing hormone levels, stress, gastro-enteritis, smoking, antibiotics, certain foods (such as dairy foods, starches or alcohol), excessive exercise or pelvic surgery.

Women are twice as likely as men to suffer from IBS and women with IBS are more likely than the average woman to have back pain, heavy or painful periods, pain during sex, cystitis, headaches, tiredness and depression.

what to do yourself

Exercise – Take regular whole-body exercise to reduce your stress levels by giving you a natural 'high' and to relieve tension. Moving your body also encourages good digestion by stimulating your intestines.

Dietary changes – Counteract indigestion and avoid any foods that you know upset your bowels. Avoid added bran, and cut down on coffee, tea and cola.

Identify any food sensitivity (see page 261).

Stress management – Breathing exercises and muscle relaxation can help, and some women with IBS find meditation and yoga particularly useful.

symptom sorter

Gynae or gynae-related causes of an irritable bowel

●●● **Most likely** – certain foods, gastro-enteritis, 'stress'

●● **Less likely** – antibiotics, smoking, too much exercise, unusual sensitivity to changing sex hormone levels, endometriosis

● **Possible** – pelvic surgery

Massage and aromatherapy – Relieve emotional and physical tension with an abdominal massage, using two teaspoons of sweet almond or other carrier oil to which you've added three drops of lavender oil. (Note the cautions on page 288 when using aromatherapy oils.)

Herbal remedies – Help relax your intestines after eating by drinking a cup of peppermint, chamomile or ginger-root tea. Remedies containing artichoke leaf extract may also be useful. (Note the cautions on page 277 when using herbal remedies.)

Hydrotherapy – A comfortably hot bath may ease painful intestinal spasms.

Acupuncture – Some people find this helps to relieve symptoms.

Tests and investigations

Your doctor may want to exclude other causes of abdominal pain, such as lactose (milk sugar) intolerance, pelvic inflammatory disease and endometriosis.

need to see a doctor?

See your doctor if you pass blood or if your pain or 'bowel habit' are different from usual

Medical treatment

Once IBS is confirmed, you may – depending on your symptoms – benefit from drugs to calm your bowel, or to encourage more frequent bowel motions

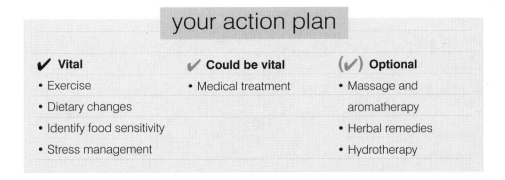

your action plan

✔ **Vital**	✔ **Could be vital**	(✔) **Optional**
• Exercise	• Medical treatment	• Massage and aromatherapy
• Dietary changes		
• Identify food sensitivity		• Herbal remedies
• Stress management		• Hydrotherapy

other conditions with gynae links

This section outlines the gynae links of certain other conditions.

acne

This can result from oversensitivity to normal levels of testosterone and is common in teenagers. Most grow out of it within five years but in more than one in 20 it persists, or reappears later. Acne increases sebum (skin oil) production, alters its nature and makes hair-follicle lining cells more sticky. This can block follicles and encourage infection by bacteria normally present on skin. Oxygen in the air causes a chemical change (oxidation) in the oils in the dammed-up sebum and turns it black, producing blackheads.

Acne is a common feature of polycystic ovary syndrome (PCOS). Other triggers include a falling oestrogen level pre-menstrually, the progestogen-only Pill, high humidity, stress and certain drugs.

asthma

Asthma inflames the airways and makes them unusually sensitive to certain triggers, causing their lining to swell and produce mucus and their muscles to tighten. All this narrows them, causing a cough, wheezing and tight chest.

In childhood boys are more asthma-prone than are girls but the numbers equalise in the teens and from the age of 20 until after the menopause women have more asthma, partly because of hormone changes during periods and pregnancy. Later, the tables turn again. Around a third of women with asthma find its severity changes with their menstrual cycle, though the Pill can smooth out such changes. During pregnancy one in three women with asthma has more trouble from it, one in three has less and in the rest there is no change. A woman whose unborn baby is a girl may have more worsening of asthma than one whose baby is a boy. Around the menopause women are four times more likely than at other times to need in-patient hospital care for asthma.

Other possible triggers include cold air, exercise, laughter, infection, smoke, fumes from poorly maintained gas appliances, vehicle fumes, stress, perfume, airborne chemicals from new clothes, paint, glue, shoe waterproofing or conditioning spray, a sudden fall in air-pressure and thunderstorms. Another possibility is allergy – to certain foods (such as peanuts, oranges, milk, eggs), drugs (for example, aspirin), food additives, house-dust mites, pollens, moulds, food mites or animal dander (skin flakes, etc, from the coat). Also, hyperventilation encourages symptoms and asthma can run in families.

autoimmune diseases

Our immune system helps to protect us from infecting organisms, foreign particles and cancer cells. Sometimes, though, immune cells 'change sides' and attack our cells as if these were invaders. This mistake results from a mutation of antibodies known as antigen-receptors that are embedded in immune cells and are normally protective. Generally, if an immune cell has mutated antibodies, it self-destructs but if the immune system isn't working properly, such cells can attack normal tissue and cause autoimmune ('self-allergic') disease. The cause isn't clear but it's thought that anything that reduces immunity may play a part – including stress, a poor diet, an inflamed gut, a lack of exercise and too much sunshine. There are many autoimmune diseases and most are more likely after a premature or early menopause.

Rheumatoid arthritis (RA) is one example and young women are particularly prone to it. The Pill lowers the risk, childlessness increases it and some people inherit a high risk. Pregnancy can improve RA up until three months after childbirth. Another example is lupus, which can be associated with frequent miscarriage due to blood clots within the placenta, arthritis, skin rashes and kidney damage. Others autoimmune diseases include type 1 diabetes, Hashimoto's thyroiditis, systemic sclerosis (thickening and tightening of connective tissue), Sjögren's syndrome (see pages 174-177), glomerulonephritis (a type of kidney inflammation) and AIDS (see page 213).

It's possible that autoimmune attack may also cause endometriosis and unexplained ovarian failure before the age of 40 (page 221).

chronic fatigue syndrome

If tiredness or exhaustion continue for weeks and are combined with certain other symptoms (such as headaches, aching muscles, poor memory, sore throat, and poor sleep) and if your doctor finds no obvious cause, you almost certainly have CFS/ME (chronic fatigue syndrome/myalgic encephalomyelitis). This cumbersome label – which is under review – isn't attached until fatigue has lasted for at least six months. CFS/ME is twice as common in women as it is in men and it encourages pelvic pain.

No one knows its cause, but experts suspect that several small changes in the levels or actions of immune factors, hormones, and neurotransmitters have a disabling effect. Possible triggers include stress, allergy and viral infection. People with depression, fibromyalgia, or irritable bowel syndrome have an increased risk. There are no specific tests or investigations. Most people improve in time and it's best to start treatment early.

gluten sensitivity (intolerance)

A slow-onset immune reaction to gluten-containing food triggers the production of antibodies to gluten (a protein in wheat, barley and rye). These damage the bowel and can cause coeliac disease (diarrhoea, stomach ache, wind and weight loss). They can also enter the blood and be deposited elsewhere, encouraging irregular periods, miscarriage, infertility, osteoporosis, depression, nerve disorders, seizures, blisters, mouth ulcers, pitted, discoloured teeth and bowel cancer. Gluten-sensitive ulcers are more likely before a period when hormone changes lower immunity and make mucus less protective.

If a blood test for gluten antibodies is positive you need a gut biopsy. This is because gluten encourages bowel cancer and lymphoma in gluten-sensitive people and the treatment for gluten sensitivity is avoiding wheat, barley and rye for life. However, you should not enter into such a commitment without definite evidence of gut damage. You can replace foods made from gluten-containing grains with foods made from other grains, such as rice, corn, buckwheat and quinoa. For years gluten-sensitive people have been advised not to eat oats, as these contain a protein similar to gluten. However, when Finnish researchers examined bowel biopsies from 63 people with coeliac disease after five years on a gluten-free diet, the gut lining in those who went on eating oats was as healthy as that in those who abstained. So they concluded it's safe to eat oats in moderation.

joint and muscle problems

Breast infections, sexually transmitted infections and pelvic inflammatory disease can make joints and muscles ache. A Norwegian study has found a strong association between certain joint and muscle conditions and the likelihood of a gynae disease, particularly for women with fibromyalgia, whiplash injury (due to a sudden jerking of the neck) or arthritis – all of whom were significantly more likely to have period problems, long-term pelvic pain and pelvic inflammatory disease.

Fibromyalgia refers to muscle pains and stiffness, often with 'knots' and 'cords' in the shoulders and back and tenderness in many points in the neck, chest, elbow, buttock or knee. Other names for this are muscular rheumatism and fibrositis. It sometimes begins after a shock and therefore increased sensitivity to pain and a low level of the neurotransmitter serotonin may be partly responsible.

Most people with fibromyalgia are women and up to nine in 10 have a disturbed sleep pattern. Their activity level, stress and the weather may also affect symptoms. Several other conditions are likely to accompany fibromyalgia – including headaches, Raynaud's phenomenon, poor memory or concentration, depression, restless legs, and irritable bowel syndrome.

migraine

Gynae triggers include premenstrual hormone changes and the Pill. (Other triggers include stress, bright or flashing lights, loud noise, certain weather conditions, hunger and food sensitivity – most often to cheese, milk, oranges, alcohol or wheat).

overactive thyroid

An overactive thyroid causes sweating, heat, hunger, shaky hands and a rapid or irregular heartbeat. The thyroid may swell and you may feel anxious, restless and tired. You may have scanty, irregular periods and fertility problems. Sleep may become difficult. You may also have itching, weight loss, diarrhoea, irritability and incontinence. Sometimes there is swelling of the front of the lower leg, plus a rash there. Three in five people suffer from muscle wasting, weakness, stiffness and cramps. And one person in 10 develops eye problems due to inflammation in the muscles and fat around the eyes – sometimes years before or after other symptoms.

The most common cause of thyroid overactivity (thyrotoxicosis) is autoimmune antibody attack (Graves' disease), which mostly affects young and middle-aged women. The trigger is unclear, though stress may play a part.

Thyroid overactivity can run in families; other causes include pregnancy, inflammation, infection, a thyroid or pituitary tumour and certain drugs.

underactive thyroid

The thyroid gland, located in the front of the neck, produces two hormones under the control of the pituitary and hypothalamus. These hormones help to regulate body growth and both cellular oxygen consumption and heat production. One in 10 women has an underactive thyroid at some time and women are ten times more likely than men to have this condition. Indeed, the American Thyroid Association has called for thyroid hormone screening to be begun at the age of 35 and believes this is especially important for women.

An underactive thyroid can cause heavy periods, fertility problems, fatigue, weak, aching muscles, coldness and weight gain. The skin may be dry and pale, with puffiness around the eyes. Some women develop anaemia, constipation, bloating, swollen ankles and depression. A croaky voice, unsteadiness and insomnia are also possible, while numb and tingling fingers, rheumatoid arthritis and heart disease are more common and the gland can swell. Too low a level of thyroid hormones can increase prolactin production (see Nipple itching and/or discharge, page 70).

Triggers include autoimmune antibody attack (Hashimoto's thyroiditis), a poor diet, treatment for an overactive thyroid and certain drugs. An underactive thyroid after childbirth can mimic postnatal depression. Smoking, stress and inactivity may reduce thyroid hormone levels too.

part three / natural cures

Here we'll look more closely at some of the lifestyle tips and other self-help treatments recommended earlier. These include details on foods rich in particular nutrients; the glycaemic index of certain foods; food sensitivity; aerobic, pelvic floor and pelvic tilt exercises and various forms of light and stress management. There is also practical information about herbal remedies and essential oils.

a healthy diet

A healthy diet is one that maintains a healthy weight and has a good balance of the major nutrients – protein, fats and carbohydrates – plus enough vitamins, minerals, and plant pigments and hormones to optimise health.

Each day aim to eat:

• At least three, preferably more, helpings of vegetables, including at least one helping of salad or other raw vegetables.

• At least two helpings of fruit – favouring whole fruit, although one helping can be a glass of fruit juice.

• Several helpings of complex carbohydrates – including starches (in root vegetables, rice, and cereal-grain foods made from wheat, oats, barley, rye, corn), and fibre (now known as non-starch polysaccharides and not absorbed but vital for health; in wholegrain-cereal foods, brown rice and all vegetables and fruit).

• Moderate amounts of animal and/or vegetable protein (in meat, fish, eggs, milk, cheese, yoghurt, peas, beans and bean products such as tofu).

• A little fat – to provide less than a third of your daily calories. Over two-thirds of your calories from fat should come from unsaturated fats – including monounsaturated fats (in avocados; olives, almonds, hazelnuts, peanuts and sesame seeds and their oils) and polyunsaturated fats (omega-6 and omega-3 fatty acids – see page 256). The rest of your calories from fat can come from saturated fats (in fatty meat, eggs, dairy products, most margarine, white cooking fat, and coconut oil).

And several times a week aim to eat:

• A helping of beans, peas or other foods rich in plant oestrogens (see page 260).

• A helping of oily fish (such as salmon, mackerel, herring, sardines, pilchards);if you dislike fish, eat other foods rich in omega-3s (see page 256).

foods, nutrients and gynae disorders

Some home treatments involve eating more foods rich in particular nutrients. This section helps you to decide which to choose and also tells you which disorders are particularly likely to be helped by each nutrient. It also includes lists of foods rich in plant pigments and plant oestrogens and foods with a low or high glycaemic index.

omega-3 and omega-6 fatty acids

These two groups of fatty acids are vital for good immunity and a good balance of hormones, prostaglandins and neurotransmitters. One of each group is essential: alpha-linolenic acid is the essential omega-3 fatty acid and linoleic acid is the essential omega-6. If your food contains enough of these two your body can normally make enough of all the others.

However, many people eat too many foods rich in omega-6s and not enough rich in omega-3s. Also, stress or ageing may prevent the conversion of alpha-linolenic and linoleic acids to other omega-3s and omega-6s. Many gynae problems can occur as a result.

A good balance is particularly helpful for: breast pain, breast cancer, period pain, heavy periods, premenstrual syndrome, endometriosis, infertility, fibroids, inflamed Bartholin's gland, dry vulva and vagina, sexually transmitted infections, leaking of urine, bingeing, lactose intolerance.

other healthy-diet tips

- When eating foods made from grains, favour wholegrain rather than refined-grain varieties. For example, choose wholegrain or wholemeal bread rather than white or brown and brown rice rather than white.

- Keep foods containing added sugar to a minimum.

- Use rapeseed (canola) oil for frying but avoid too much fried food.

- Favour low-GI foods (see below) and home-prepared whole foods.

- Check the contents of commercially processed foods, as many contain a lot of fat, salt and sugar.

Sources of omega-3s include: green-leafy vegetables, broccoli, beans and bean products (such as tofu), walnuts and their oil, pumpkin seeds, linseeds (flaxseeds; the richest source), wholegrain-cereal foods, rapeseed (canola) and soybean oils, meat from grass-fed animals, oily fish.

Sources of omega-6s include: avocados; beans; corn; seeds; sunflower-seed, safflower, sesame, peanut (groundnut), corn and soybean oils; wholegrain-cereal foods.

vitamins

Beta-carotene ('pro-vitamin A')

The body converts this carotenoid plant pigment into vitamin A.

Particularly helpful for: breast pain, cancer, heavy or irregular periods, premenstrual syndrome, endometriosis, fibroids, dry vulva and vagina, inflamed Bartholin's gland, candida, pelvic inflammatory disease, sexually transmitted infections, cystitis, overweight.

Sources include: orange, red and dark green fruits and vegetables.

Vitamin B

Particularly helpful for: breast pain; cancer; painful, irregular, absent or scanty periods; endometriosis; infertility; fibroids; cervical erosion; dry vulva and vagina (B6); low sex drive; bingeing.

One B vitamin, folic acid, may be particularly helpful for breast and cervix cancer, infertility, and sexually transmitted infections.

Sources include:

Vitamin B – meat, fish, dairy produce, eggs, beans, peas, green leafy vegetables, mushrooms, nuts, seeds, wholegrain foods.

Vitamin B6 – beans, peas, green leafy vegetables, mushrooms, nuts, seeds, wholegrain foods.

Folic acid – dairy produce, eggs, nuts, fruits, vegetables (especially green leafy), beans, peas, whole grains.

Inositol – eggs, liver, citrus fruit, beans, wholegrain foods.

Vitamin C

Particularly helpful for: cancer, painful or heavy periods, premenstrual syndrome, endometriosis, infertility, fibroids, prolapse, inflamed Bartholin's gland, dry vulva and vagina, candida, pelvic inflammatory disease, sexually transmitted infections, cystitis, osteoporosis, overweight, bingeing.

Sources include: fruit and vegetables.

Vitamin E

Particularly helpful for: fungal skin infections; cancer; period pain; irregular, absent or scanty periods; premenstrual syndrome; endometriosis; infertility; fibroids; inflamed Bartholin's gland; dry vulva and vagina; candida; pelvic inflammatory disease; low sex drive; sexually transmitted infections; overweight.

Sources include: meat, fish, dairy produce, eggs, green leafy vegetables, beans, peas, sweet potatoes, mangoes, nuts, seeds, wholegrain foods.

minerals

Calcium

Particularly helpful for: breast cancer, period pain, heavy periods, premenstrual syndrome, prolapse, osteoporosis, bingeing.

Sources include: tinned fish eaten with their bones, shellfish, dairy produce, eggs, beans, peas, lentils, nuts, seeds, wholegrain foods.

Iron

Particularly helpful for: heavy periods, anaemia.

Sources include: meat (including liver), shellfish, eggs, green leafy vegetables, elderberries, beans, peas, nuts, seeds, wholegrain foods.

Magnesium

Particularly helpful for: period pain, heavy periods, endometriosis, polycystic ovary syndrome, fibroids, osteoporosis, bingeing.

Sources include: meat, fish, eggs, green leafy vegetables, mushrooms, beans, peas, nuts, seeds, wholegrain foods.

Selenium

Particularly helpful for: cancer, endometriosis, infertility, inflamed Bartholin's gland, candida, pelvic inflammatory disease, sexually transmitted infections, overweight.

Sources include: meat, fish, dairy produce, eggs, green leafy vegetables, mushrooms, garlic, beans, peas, wholegrain foods.

Zinc

Particularly helpful for: cancer, heavy periods, endometriosis, infertility, polycystic ovary syndrome, candida, pelvic inflammatory disease, low sex drive, sexually transmitted infections, cystitis, osteoporosis, overweight, bingeing.

Sources include: meat, dairy produce, fish, shellfish, root vegetables, beans, peas, garlic, nuts, seeds, wholegrain foods.

Fibre

Particularly helpful for: lumpy or painful breasts, cancer, heavy or irregular periods, endometriosis, fibroids, polycystic ovary syndrome, infertility.

Sources include: fruits, vegetables, wholegrain foods.

antioxidants

These include beta-carotene, vitamins C and E, selenium, zinc, plant pigments, inositol (see vitamin B) and substances in spices (such as curcumin in turmeric and mustard, and shogaols, gingerols and zingiberene in ginger). Interestingly, many plant oestrogens are antioxidants too. See separate entries for information on what each is particularly helpful for.

plant pigments

These important antioxidants are present in all brightly coloured fruits and vegetables.

Particularly helpful for: cancer, heavy periods, endometriosis, prolapse, inflamed Bartholin's gland, pelvic inflammatory disease, sexually transmitted infections, osteoporosis, overweight, cystitis.

Flavonoids

Quercetin, rutin, curcumin, polyphenols (including tannins such as proanthocyanidins), resveratrol, genistein, tangeretin, nobiletin, catechins and oleuropein.

Sources include: blue, black and dark-red berries and cherries and grapes (for proanthocyanidins), grapes (for resveratrol), olives (for oleuropein) and onions and tea (for quercetin).

Carotenoids

Beta-carotene, lycopene (the most powerful natural antioxidant), lutein and zeaxanthin.

Sources include: carrots, apricots, melon, green leafy vegetables, sweet potatoes (for beta-carotene); egg yolk, corn, red grapes, pumpkin, orange peppers and green leafy vegetables (for lutein and zeaxanthin); tomatoes (for lycopene).

plant oestrogens

Particularly helpful for: lumpy or painful breasts; heavy or irregular periods; polycystic ovary syndrome; endometriosis; infertility; fibroids; breast; womb or ovary cancer; dry vagina; premenstrual syndrome; cervical erosion; low sex drive; menopausal flushes and sweats; leaking of urine; osteoporosis.

Sources include: aubergines, beans, peas, lentils, chick peas, celery, root vegetables, cabbage, fennel, garlic, cherries, plums, rhubarb, wholegrain foods, rice, seeds, sprouted beans and other seeds, nuts soaked in water overnight, olives, parsley, sage, turmeric, beer, wine.

bitter foods

Particularly helpful for: lumpy or painful breasts; heavy or irregular periods; polycystic ovary syndrome; endometriosis; infertility; fibroids; breast, womb and ovary cancers; cervical erosion.

Sources include: lettuce, cabbage, watercress, chicory, bean sprouts, artichokes, liver, olives, rosemary, turmeric, horseradish, dandelion tea, tonic water.

glycaemic index (gi)

This is an indicator of how fast a food raises your blood-sugar level. High-GI foods (see below) raise it fast and eating large amounts on a regular basis encourages several health problems, including diabetes. This is because high blood sugar stimulates the pancreas to release insulin, the hormone that enables sugar to enter cells and affects fat metabolism. Years of repeated over-stimulation by insulin encourages cells to resist its actions, so the pancreas has to produce much more to get sugar into cells. This is called insulin resistance – or pre-diabetes because, if it continues, the pancreas is likely to become exhausted and therefore produce very little insulin, leading to the constantly raised blood sugar of diabetes.

Most of us eat too much high-GI food, so we have a raised risk of both pre-diabetes and diabetes.

The solution is to favour low-GI foods, and when you do eat high-GI foods, to:

- eat only a small amount
- eat some low-GI food in the same meal or snack

These are particularly helpful tips for: endometriosis, polycystic ovary syndrome, overweight, bingeing.

Here are some examples of relatively low- and high-GI foods (visit www.mendosa.com/gilists.htm)/ for a more comprehensive list.)

Relatively low-GI foods include: proteins, fats, nuts, green vegetables, beans, carrots, most fruit, pearl barley, Burgen bread, pasta.

Relatively high-GI foods include: fruit canned in syrup, dates, swede, potatoes, parsnips, bread (especially baguettes), most breakfast cereals (not All-Bran), biscuits, crackers, pastry, pizza.

identifying food sensitivity

This may be helpful for: heavy periods, infertility, cystitis, migraine and perhaps even some cancers (for example, if you have gluten sensitivity, gluten encourages bowel cancer).

Food sensitivity is a condition that is frequently covered in women's magazines and popular health books. However, it is uncommon, less likely in adults than in children and it can be difficult to be sure about it – indeed, studies show that many adults who believe they are sensitive to a food are not. This can be problematic because people may cut out important foods such as wheat and milk unnecessarily. Unless they know what to eat instead to maintain a balanced diet, they could easily go short of nutrients.

If you suspect food sensitivity, don't waste your money on food-intolerance tests, as the only way to be sure is to do a food-elimination and multiple-challenge test. Talk to a doctor or dietician if you don't know how to keep your diet healthy when you cut out a staple (such as wheat or milk) or if you are dealing with a child or someone who is unwell. **Note:** if you've ever had an allergic response to a food, such as urticaria (nettle rash or hives), swollen lips or throat, or breathing difficulty, it is *essential* that any challenge tests you undertake are medically supervised.

Food-elimination and multiple-challenge test.

Test one food at a time. To prove sensitivity to that food, three challenges must be positive. This test can help identify food sensitivity as a cause of readily reversilbe conditions such as cystitis and migraine.

1.   Avoid the suspect for three weeks. If your symptoms settle it may or may not be because you were sensitive to it. So, to challenge your suspicion, eat it again; if your symptoms return this is the first positive challenge. (Out of interest, take your pulse before and after eating the suspect; a rise of more than 10 beats a minute suggests sensitivity.)

2.   Stop eating the food for a week, then try it again. If your symptoms return this is the second positive challenge.

3.   Stop eating the food for a further week, then try it again. If your symptoms return this is the third positive challenge.

To identify food sensitivity as a cause of heavy periods, avoid the food for a month at a time before each challenge.

Even if three challenges are positive you may find you can eat the food in question in small amounts or less frequently. Alternatively, you may have to avoid it entirely. If you are sensitive to cereal grains or milk tell your doctor, as you may need specific tests for lactose intolerance or gluten sensitivity.

exercise

Each of the three main sorts of exercise – aerobic, strengthening (strength or endurance) and stretching (flexibility) – is beneficial for almost every gynae disorder.

General advice

• If you are unfit – and especially if you have high blood pressure, diabetes or heart disease – check with your doctor before embarking on a fitness programme.

• Start by warming up, for example with marching or low-impact jogging. Warm muscles are more flexible and less prone to stiffening after exercise. Don't strip off until you feel warm.

• Stretch each muscle group before aerobic or strengthening exercise, to help prevent damage from sudden movements of tense muscles.

• Gradually wind down your exercise level towards the end of aerobic or strengthening exercise, stretch again after exercising and keep warm.

• Drink little and often. For example, drink half a glass of water before a 30-60 minute session of aerobic or strengthening exercise, then another half-glass every 20 minutes. For a longer session prepare a drink containing half fruit juice, half water and a small pinch of salt in each half pint. Commercial sports drinks are expensive and sugary, so you might want to avoid them. Restore energy with a banana every hour or so.

• Don't give up exercising if you get bored. Instead, copy successful long-term exercisers by choosing something that is more appealing or fits in better with your personality or lifestyle. And if you're bored with an instructor, work with another one or suggest changes.

Aerobic exercise

This involves brisk movements that boost your circulation and make you feel warmer and breathe faster. Aerobic exercise is important for the following reasons:

• It raises the rate at which cells burn energy (the metabolic rate); you also burn an extra 200-300 calories a day for 24-48 hours after exercise, which helps you shed excess fat or lets you eat more without gaining weight.

- It increases the circulation throughout your whole body, including your sex-hormone glands and sex organs.

- It helps balance hormones in general, as well as neurotransmitters.

- It boosts fertility and immunity.

- It helps to counteract stress and prevent fluid retention – including pelvic congestion.

- It raises the levels of endorphins, which lifts spirits, increases vitality, wellbeing and *joie de vivre* and makes any pain easier to tolerate.

'Aerobic' exercise is so called because the muscle cells receive all the oxygen they need. If you exercise so fast or hard that muscles hurt, you are no longer exercising aerobically – the pain warns of a shortage of oxygen and a build-up of lactic acid.

Even gentle aerobic exercise, such as a leisurely walk, or swim, is good for health. But to benefit your heart and circulation and burn fat, you need to increase your heart rate to the 'cardiovascular' or 'cardio' range. This might mean doing such things as fast walking, gentle, low-impact jogging, or brisk swimming. Moderate-intensity cardio work is exercise vigorous enough to raise your heart rate to 50-75 per cent of its safe maximum rate. The absolute maximum that's safe for the human heart is 220 beats each minute, and *your* safe maximum depends on your age.

To work out 50-75 per cent of your safe maximum heart rate:

- Subtract your age from 220 – for your safe maximum.

- Multiply this figure by 0.75 for your upper cardio limit.

- Multiply the same figure by 0.5 for your lower cardio limit.

working out your cardio range

For example, **for a woman aged 30**, her safe maximum is 220-30 = 190.

Her lower cardio limit is 50 per cent of 190 = 95.

And her upper cardio limit is 75 per cent of 190 = 142.5 – say 142.

Her cardio range is therefore 95–142 beats a minute.

Aim to get slightly breathless, so that you can hear yourself breathing but can still talk.

How much do you need? Do at least half an hour of aerobic exercise on at least five days of the week. It can be either low-intensity (such as walking or gardening) or moderate-intensity (such as brisk walking, dancing, jogging, cycling or swimming). It's fine to split the half-hour into several shorter sessions. Ideally three of these sessions should involve 30-60 minutes of cardio exercise.

Muscle-strengthening

This involves moving your muscles against resistance, to make them work harder. This makes them bigger, which means they are more powerful and can burn up more fat. Examples include carrying or lifting any weight (such as a young child or backpack), digging and cycling uphill.

How much do you need? Do some muscle-strengthening exercise preferably every other day, but at least twice a week.

Stretching

This elongates muscles. It may be that first luxurious early morning stretch, a part of everyday activities (such as reaching for things on high shelves), or as part of scheduled exercise (such as aerobic, dance and yoga classes, or tennis or swimming). A good stretch helps after staying in one position a long time, such as when sitting at a desk or lying in bed. Stretching helps to:

- prevent muscles from gradually becoming shorter and less flexible

- prevent inactive muscles, tendons and joints from stiffening

- relieve aching from muscle tension

- improve balance and posture

- make you feel brighter and more energetic.

How much do you need? Do some stretching every day.

Pelvic floor (Kegel) exercises.

This can be helpful for: dry vagina and vulva, low sex drive, leaking of urine, prolapse, pelvic inflammatory disease, sexually transmitted infections.

pelvic floor exercises

First, learn to recognise the muscles by feeling them tighten when you interrupt the flow of urine, tighten your vagina around one or two fingers (or a tampon or partner's penis), and stop yourself passing wind.

Do a set of exercises five times a day, sitting or lying with knees slightly apart.

For each set, tighten the muscles for two seconds, then relax for two, and repeat 10 times.

Over two weeks, work up to 10 seconds' tightening and 10 seconds' relaxing. Aim to relax for an increasingly short time as your pelvic floor gets fitter.

Pelvic floor exercises work the 'pelvic-floor muscles' – the pubococcygeal muscles in the pelvic floor. This is a muscular 'hammock' that's normally strong and elastic enough to support the bladder, urethra, womb and rectum.

Pelvic rocking

This can be helpful for: period pain, pelvic inflammatory disease.

Pelvic rocking involves kneeling on all fours and moving your lower back with repeated little up and down movements for a minute several times a day or as necessary.

stress management

This can be helpful for: any stressful gynae disorder and any gynae disorder exacerbated by stress.

Stress influences every part of our body via its effects on our hormones, neurotransmitters and immunity and too much stress can have profound effects on our health. It can make us feel tired, irritable, anxious or depressed. It can trigger headaches, 'butterflies' in the stomach, 'nervous diarrhoea', sweating, shaking and hyperventilation and cause dizziness, phobias and panic attacks. It can encourage addictive behaviours – such as out of control drinking, smoking, sex, work, shopping, gambling and exercise. It can also be at the root of eating disorders, reduce immunity and spark off illnesses such as asthma and irritable bowel syndrome. Stress that continues for weeks or months encourages many gynae disorders (including period problems and infertility) and worsens many others (including pelvic pain, low sex drive, and menopausal flushes).

The most likely causes of stress are work or family problems; anything that makes you angry, frustrated, fearful or jealous; pain and illness. Too much caffeine raises stress hormone levels; some foods encourage anxiety by changing the levels of certain hormones and neurotransmitters and eating too few foods containing calcium, magnesium and vitamins E and B (needed for healthy nerves) can be to blame. A low blood sugar level can provoke anxiety: some people – especially those who are overweight, eat badly and don't exercise enough – sometimes have this problem between meals because their cells don't repond normally to insulin; this is called 'insulin resistance' or 'pre-diabetes' (see page 261). Other causes of low blood sugar to consider include too much alcohol on an empty stomach, poorly treated diabetes, and certain cancers and pituitary or liver disorders.

Depression is another common anxiety trigger; indeed, anxiety and depression very often occur together. Its possible causes include shock, loss, suppressed emotion, hormone changes, lack of bright light, poor diet and physical inactivity. Sometimes there's no apparent cause.

Smoking can be stressful too, for while some people turn to cigarettes to relieve stress, smoking actually raises the adrenaline level. Other causes of stress include hyperventilation ('overbreathing' – breathing too much air, whether rapidly, deeply or shallowly, which can also cause tingling, ringing in the ears and chest pain) and an overactive thyroid. Rarely, the blame falls on an adrenal gland tumour producing a high adrenaline level. Certain slimming drugs encourage anxiety and other culprits include schizophrenia, dementia and withdrawal from high levels of alcohol or illegal drugs. Some people feel anxious only in certain situations – such as when flying, performing, doing exams or when in open spaces or at extreme heights. A panic attack may cause chest pain and breathlessness that can be confused with a heart attack; it is always best to seek help if you're unsure as to what's going on, as sudden unexplained anxiety or fear is occasionally the first sign of a heart attack.

What to do

Work out a selection of effective, non-damaging stress-management strategies to use as required. What follows are 12 practical suggestions for stressbusting, 10 suggestions for altering your mindset so you see life differently, and four important 'life skills'.

Twelve practical suggestions

1. **Aim to identify the trigger** – so that you can avoid or counteract it, if possible.

2. **See a doctor if necessary** – especially if your anxiety is severe or interferes with daily life despite home treatment. Your doctor will rule out disorders such as depression or an overactive thyroid and will help you to decide on a course of action. Some people benefit from tranquillisers for two to four weeks while they find effective long-term strategies for managing their stress. It isn't wise to take these drugs for longer, however, as they can have side effects and they can become addictive. If necessary, your doctor will recommend a counsellor or therapist.

3. **Make dietary changes** – Eat a healthy diet with regular meals and try to include some naturally calming foods that are rich in unrefined carbohydrate, vitamins B and E, calcium and magnesium (see page 257). Steady your blood sugar by eating mainly low-GI foods (see page 261). High-carbohydrate, low-protein snacks are useful between meals as they contain an amino acid called tryptophan which will help to boost your serotonin level; examples include wholemeal bread, bananas, dates, hazelnuts, pumpkin seeds, and beans.

4. **Avoid too much caffeine** – especially at night, when it can keep you awake, worrying.

5. **Take exercise** – Stretch to ease muscle tension and take some brisk exercise to boost your levels of 'feel-good' endorphins (see page 263) and burn off high levels of stress hormones.

6. **Get more exposure to light** – Go outside in bright daylight for at least half an hour a day to raise your level of serotonin. Consider using a light visor or box, or wearing a flashing-light mask, for a while each day (see also page 291 and Helplist, page 315).

7. **Have a massage** – Try having a massage – or even giving one, which some people find just as relaxing.

8. **Use aromatherapy** – Add a few drops of 'calming' oils such as lavender to your bath water, or add them to a carrier oil for a massage. (Note the cautions on page 288 when using aromatherapy oils.)

9. **Use hydrotherapy** – Relax in a comfortably hot, scented bath, perhaps with candlelight, soft music and a book or magazine.

10. **Try herbal remedies** – Drink a cup of chamomile, lime (linden) blossom or lemon balm tea several times a day.

11. **Adjust breathing** – Taking a few slow breaths can be excellent 'first aid' if you're feeling stressed. If you feel panicky, you may be hyperventilating; try breathing into a paper bag, or your cupped hands, for two minutes, then concentrate on breathing more slowly and normally. Exercise will also help you feel better, though is best avoided if you are feeling faint as well as panicky.

12. **Boost wellbeing** – Do at least one enjoyable, relaxing or sybaritic activity each day, then double its benefits by thinking about it afterwards. Also, create opportunities to have fun or a good laugh – even when you don't feel like it.

Ten suggestions to help you see life differently

1. **See stressful situations as challenges** – Look at each stressful situation as a challenge rather than a hardship, then formulate suitable tactics, set goals, evaluate progress regularly and use new tactics if necessary.

2. **Boost your self-esteem** – Do this whenever times are tough by reminding yourself of your good qualities.

3. **Pray or meditate.**

4. **Deal with challenging emotions** – such as anger and fear, by recognising and naming them and then either expressing them (if safe and appropriate) or channelling their energy into more creative or community-building pursuits.

5. **Get professional help** – if necessary, with health, relationships, finances, business affairs or addictive habits. The latter may seem to help you cope with stress but they actually damage you (or others), especially in the long-term. Such habits can include eating or drinking too much, eating too little, smoking, having affairs, being a workaholic, avoiding work, shopping compulsively, taking recreational drugs and driving too fast.

6. **Change your perspective** – for example, reflect on what really matters: are your expectations realistic? Are you doing – as far as possible – what you want? Challenge all the 'shoulds', 'oughts' and 'musts'. Learn to let yourself and others make mistakes. And remember that bad times invariably do pass.

7. **Say 'No' sometimes** – when you are overstretched, and learn to delegate without feeling guilty. Practise prioritising too (meaning doing the most important things first).

8. **Set yourself realistic deadlines.**

9. **Be assertive** – Let others know what you want or what you think without putting them down or being aggressive.

10. **Use the 'Anxiety' tips** on page 268.

Four important 'life skills' for your stress-management portfolio

1. Being a good listener

This means listening empathically so that you recognise and acknowledge the emotions that often lie behind words. Listening in this way to yourself helps you to be more aware of your own real needs and feelings. Listening in this way to others helps you to get to know them better, and helps them to feel heard and understood.

When listening to yourself, simply aim to recognise and name your emotions, both obvious and underlying. When listening to others:

a. Put *your* emotions to one side for the time being.

b. Recognise and name their emotions. These may not be obvious, but you'll find clues in what they say and how they say it and in their body language.

c. Say what you think they may be feeling – for example, 'It seems to me you're feeling XXX' or 'It sounds as if you're feeling XXX …'. If you're wrong they won't mind and will soon put you right. And whether you're right or wrong, you'll start them thinking.

2. Dealing well with disagreement

Disagreements, arguments and strife are a natural part of relating but can be associated with huge amounts of emotion. Conflict resolution skills help prevent emotions such as anger from doing damage.

There are six steps:

a. Decide who needs to talk – or, more exactly, *be heard* – first.

b. Agree that you will both aim to listen empathically when it's your turn to listen.

c. When it's your turn to talk say '*I* feel', not '*You make me* feel'.

d. Take turns at listening and talking until you both feel heard and understood. The conflict may not yet at this point be resolved but you now have a good basis for further discussion. Recognising how someone feels doesn't mean you agree with their position but it does mean that you've tried to understand how they feel, which is vitally important.

e. Brainstorm ways of moving forward.

f. Even if the above steps have not yet resolved the conflict, take heart from the fact that you are at least working on it together.

3. Being encouraging

This means noticing what someone is trying to do, describing it, then recognising and naming the positive feelings they get from their endeavour. Encouraging others may help them to learn to encourage you. And you can encourage yourself regularly too.

4. Imagining – or 'visualising'

This means taking time to imagine intensely beautiful or personally important situations. Many people find that this can be healing to their body, mind and spirit. The symbolic power of imagined scenes can be emotionally and spiritually significant, and help to rebalance any disturbance of neurotransmitters, hormones, 'feel-good' endorphins and immune system factors.

Here are some ideas:

• When you are unwell imagine that your healthy cells are energising and healing your unhealthy ones.

• When you pray or meditate imagine yourself receiving – or giving – love, encouragement and healing.

• When times are tough take 10-20 minutes a day to think of scenes, people or things you love or find beautiful, inspiring or healing. You might want to use the 'visualisation' overleaf.

getting stuck

Getting stuck

Anita and Jeff are at loggerheads over their spare time. They have only
recently moved in together and, whereas Anita hopes to spend much of
their free time together, Jeff has other ideas. He wants to play football on
Saturday afternoon and spend the evening with his mates on the team
afterwards and he wants to have a drink and, perhaps, a curry after work
several nights a week.

Anita says, 'You don't love me.' Jeff says, 'You make me feel hemmed in.'
These accusations make Anita feel hurt and Jeff frustrated and aching to
get out.

Last Sunday they had a row and spent the day apart. They are both so
aggrieved they are thinking of splitting up.

Moving forward

Anita and Jeff talk about how they like to spend their spare time.

Anita says, 'I like company – partly because I don't want to be on my own
like I was so much as a child – and I especially like being with you.' Jeff
says, 'I love being with you too but I need exercise, not least because I'll
put on weight like my Dad if I don't get it. I also think having a drink with
my boss after work will help me with promotion.'

Anita talks about her experience of loneliness and Jeff talks of his anxiety
about his father's health and his ambition to do well at work so they could
more easily afford to have a family. Understanding where each is coming
from makes them want to find solutions. Jeff will play football and Anita
will join him at the clubhouse. Jeff will have a drink after work once a week
and Anita will have a hen night. And Jeff is going to his boss outright
about getting more training and going for promotion.

sample visualisation

A moorland walk

Picture yourself walking along a grassy path, you see rolling moorland all around and far-off hazy mountains painting the horizon. It is early summer. The heather moors are carpeted in purples, mauves and pinks and plump blueberries burst with goodness in your mouth. Deer graze on a distant mound and swallows swoop in the sky. The golden morning sun climbs higher, its warmth enfolds your body and the scent of the land brings calm and delight. It is the start of a new day and the first day of the rest of your life.

You know you are very welcome.

Stretch your arms out wide above your head. Feel the soft spring of the earth beneath your feet and draw the moorland air deep into your lungs. Sense it energising your whole body – your legs and arms, your breasts, abdomen and pelvis, your head and back.

Now walk on, hearing the high notes of the birdsong and the deep gurgle of a moorland spring's peaty brown water. Feel the excitement, the promise and the beauty of the day. And, if you can, let your heart sing with inspiration and hope.

Tell yourself, 'I am a "child of the universe", a child of God. And, deep in my soul, I know that "all will be well … and all will be well … and all manner of things will be well".'

heat, cold and hydrotherapy

Using something hot or cold on a part of your body, such as your lower abdomen, or vulva, is an age-old way of treating gynae disorders. One readily available means of doing this is with water.

Bathing

Relaxing in a comfortably hot bath (90-95ºF) can counteract the stress of any gynae disorder and help to ease those gynae or gynae-related disorders (such as period problems and irritable bowel syndrome) that can be encouraged by stress. Try to submerge the whole of your pelvis and lower abdomen in the water and, depending on what's wrong, consider adding certain herbs, aromatherapy oils or salt to the water to counteract infection or other inflammation.

Caution: If you have high blood pressure, an itchy vulva or are pregnant, use warm water instead.

Hot/cold showers

Showering with alternately hot and cold water (use the cold for a shorter time) boosts the circulation to your whole body and therefore your pelvis too. This is good for many gynae disorders.

Contrast sitz ('sitting') bath – or hot and cold 'bum' bath

Particularly helpful for: fibroids, inflamed Bartholin's gland, cervix cell abnormalities, low sex drive, dry vagina and vulva, pelvic inflammatory disease, pelvic pain, leaking of urine.

This helps by giving your pelvic circulation a boost. Sit in hot water (105-115°F), for 3-5 minutes, then in cold (55-85°F) for 1-2 minutes, then repeat this 3-5 times, ending with cold water. If you're agile, you can organise a contrast sitz bath at home (see overleaf).

Caution: Use warm water if you have high blood pressure, an itchy vulva or are pregnant.

Hot bath/cold towel method

This method may be used as an alternative to a contrast sitz bath. Soak a large towel in cold water, then put it on the side of your bath. Sit in a hot bath for 3-5 minutes, than get out and wrap the cold wet towel around your lower abdomen and between your legs for 1-2 minutes. Repeat 3-5 times, refreshing the towel with cold water each time.

herbal remedies

Herbal remedies are an age-old way of treating gynae disorders. Most herbs contain a wide variety of active ingredients that often work together and tend to be gentler than drugs. Trained herbalists may use several herbs to treat an ailment, making their choice based on the relevant disorder's symptoms and causes. Knowing the healing actions and properties of different herbs is useful when trying herbal remedies at home.

organising a contrast sitz bath at home

Container in bath. You need a wide bath, and a large plastic container. This needs to be big enough for you to sit in and immerse your whole bottom, but no longer than half the length of the bath.

Put the container at the tap end of the bath, fill it half full with cold water, then pull it a few inches away from the taps. Fill the bath with hot water, ensuring that the water level is not so high that it will overflow into the container when you get in.

Sit in the bath water for 3-5 minutes, then get up, turn around, and sit in the container for 1-2 minutes. Repeat 3-5 times.

Or container on floor. As above, only you put the container on the floor near the bath, and fill it half full with cold water (using the bath's shower attachment makes this easier). Fill the bath with hot water.

Sit first in the bath, then in the container. Repeat 3-5 times

• When sitting in the container or bath, aim to keep your feet out of water, and put a towel around your shoulders to keep warm if necessary.

A herb's actions may be:

Anti-inflammatory

e.g. Anemone pulsatilla, arnica, black cohosh, calendula, dandelion, dong quai, feverfew, ginger, goldenseal, horsetail, juniper, lady's mantle, parsley, sage, skullcap, St John's wort, *uva ursi*, wild yam, yarrow

Immunity-boosting

e.g. arnica, astragalus, burdock, echinacea, ginseng, sage

Anti-infective

e.g. beth root, burdock, calendula, dong quai, goldenseal, juniper, lemon balm, sage, *uva ursi*

Cancer-fighting

e.g. astragalus, burdock

Diuretic (increase urine output)

e.g. buchu, cornsilk, couch grass, dandelion, horsetail, juniper, liquorice, mugwort, parsley, partridge berry, skullcap, *uva ursi*, wild yam

Astringent (decreases heavy bleeding)

e.g. beth root, calendula, cranesbill, ginseng, goldenseal, greater periwinkle, horsetail, lady's mantle, partridge berry, sage, shepherd's purse, skullcap, St John's wort, *uva ursi*, vervain, yarrow

Stimulating or relaxing ('adaptogenic'):

e.g. ginseng, liquorice

Relaxing

e.g. skullcap, vervain

Anti-depressant

e.g. St John's wort

Anti-spasmodic (acts on muscles)

e.g. Anemone pulsatilla, calendula, dong quai, ginger, lemon balm, parsley, red clover, sage, skullcap, vervain, wild yam

Womb-stimulating (can stimulate period = 'emmenagoge')

e.g. arnica, black cohosh

Womb-relaxing

e.g. goldenseal, peppermint, vervain

Womb 'tonic' (either stimulating or relaxing)

e.g. dong quai, motherwort, partridge berry, raspberry leaf, yarrow

Oestrogenic (some because they contain active plant oestrogens, others via their hormone-balancing effects on the pituitary and hypothalamus, see above)

e.g. black cohosh, dong quai (possibly), false unicorn root, fennel, ginseng, lady's mantle, liquorice, red clover, sage, wild yam

Hormone-balancing

See box opposite.

hormone-balancing herbs

Beth root – interacts with hormone receptors in the hypothalamus and pituitary to encourage ovulation.

Black cohosh – inhibits LH; improves oestrogen/progesterone balance; has a weak oestrogen-like effect by binding to certain oestrogen receptors (the beta ones in brain, bone, ovary, heart, blood-vessel, lung and bladder cells, rather than the alpha ones in breast or womb cells).

False unicorn root – may interact with hormone receptors in the hypothalamus and pituitary to encourage ovulation and so increase progesterone production; contains plant oestrogens that can occupy oestrogen receptors in cells and therefore – depending on whether a woman's own oestrogen level is high or low – either counteract a high oestrogen level (without suppressing ovulation) or have a weak oestrogenic effect.

Paeony – thought to interact with hormone receptors in the hypothalamus and pituitary to encourage ovulation and so increase progesterone production; useful for oestrogen/progesterone hormone imbalance such as that seen with oestrogen dominance because it tends to increase a low level of either hormone without producing too much of either. This helps to normalise the balance of LH and FSH. Tends to reduce a high level of prolactin. Also tends to reduce a high level of testosterone, by aiding its conversion to oestrogen in the ovaries and body fat by aromatase.

Vitex agnus castus – reduces FSH, but can increase LH and encourage ovulation (and so increase progesterone production) and increase prolactin.

Wild yam – can reduce FSH and LH. Thought to mimic progesterone by attaching to progesterone receptor sites.

(LH = luteinising hormone; FSH = follicle-stimulating hormone)

Cautions

Herbal remedies can be powerful, and can have side effects – although these tend to be milder and less common than those of medical drugs. When choosing and using herbal remedies, bear in mind the following:

All herbs

• Tell your doctor if you are taking herbal remedies, and tell your herbalist if you are taking medical drugs, as they may be less safe if taken together.

• Avoid herbal remedies if you are pregnant – or trying to be – and while breastfeeding, unless you have professional assurance that they are safe.

Hormone-balancing or oestrogenic herbs

• It's advisable to get personal advice from a qualified herbalist.

• Avoid if you are pregnant or breastfeeding.

• Consult your doctor and a herbalist first if you are on the Pill, HRT, other hormones or tamoxifen.

• Take the herb in question for at least three months.

• Report any unexpected vaginal bleeding, pelvic pain, pain during sex, vaginal discharge, or breast lump, to your doctor.

Note: the safety of herbal remedies with oestrogenic activity is unproven in women with a personal or family history of oestrogen-sensitive cancer (such as some breast, womb, ovary and colon cancers). It's possible that such remedies are safer before the menopause (when their oestrogenic activity may help to prevent the action of a woman's own, stronger oestrogen) and less safe after (supposing they are more likely to have oestrogenic activity when a woman's own oestrogen level is low). However, several of these herbs have a long history of use – red clover, for example, has actually been used to treat breast and ovary cancer, so it would seem very unlikely that they encourage cancer and likely that they discourage it.

How to make and use herbal remedies

Most of us who use herbal remedies buy them ready-made (from certain supermarkets and pharmacies or from health shops and herbal suppliers). Depending on the particular remedy, the choice may include ready-made teabags, dried leaves, flowers, stems, roots, seeds or bark, capsules or tablets, liquid extracts and alcoholic tinctures, and creams, ointments or oils.

When using tinctures or liquid extracts, follow the dosage directions on the pack. If taking several herbs with similar actions, reduce the dose of each one.

making herbal tea

- To make tea from leaves, flowers or other soft parts, put 50g (2oz) of fresh or 25g (1oz) of dried plant material in a cup, fill with just-boiled water, cover, steep for 10 minutes and strain.

- To make tea (a 'decoction') from roots, bark or seeds, chop or crush them if possible, then put 50g (2oz) of fresh or 25g (1oz) of dried plant material in a saucepan, add two cups of water, simmer for 15 minutes and strain.

Sweeten tea if desired with a little honey or sugar

Note that one teaspoon of herb tincture has about the same strength as one strong cup of herbal tea.

You can grow your own herbs for making herbal tea. And you can add home-grown or bought, fresh or dried, herbs to your food or bath water.

When treating a gynae illness continue a herbal remedy until the symptoms go or for two weeks, unless directed otherwise, or unless the herb has an oestrogenic or hormone-balancing action (see Cautions, above).

Selected herbal remedies for gynae conditions

***Anemone pulsatilla* (*pulsatilla*, pasque flower, wind flower)**

Plant with large yellow-centred purple flower.

May help: period pain, premenstrual syndrome, pelvic inflammatory disease

Part used: aerial parts

Actions: antispasmodic, womb-stimulating

Special note: only the dried plant is used, as the fresh herb contains a poisonous glycoside (ranunculin)

Caution: do not self-prescribe as the wrong dose can inflame the stomach and cause vomiting; avoid if pregnant or breastfeeding

Arnica (*Arnica montana*, leopard's bane)

Plant with yellow daisy-like flower.

May help: infected Bartholin's gland in vulva

Part used: flowers, rhizome

Actions: anti-inflammatory, immunity-boosting

Special note: used topically

Caution: don't use if vulva skin is raw; don't take by mouth

Astragalus (*Astragalus membranaceus*, Huang Qi)

Plant with yellow pea-type flower.

May help: low sex drive

Part used: root

Actions: immunity-boosting, cancer-fighting

Special notes: often recommended for weakness or fatigue; another variety, *Astragalus oxyphysis*, contains an alkaloid, swaonsonine, which may help prevent cancer from spreading.

Beth root (*Trillium erectum, birthroot, wake Robin*)

Plant with white, pink or purple three-petalled flower.

May help: heavy periods, irregular periods, fibroids, candida, trichomonas

Part used: rhizome

Actions: anti-infective, astringent, womb tonic, hormone-balancing

Caution: Don't self-prescribe, as this herb is strong (note the hormone-balancing and oestrogenic herb cautions above)

Black cohosh (*Cimicifuga racemosa*, squawroot, bugbean, black snake root, rattleroot)

Bushy plant with tall spikes of tiny creamy-white star-shaped flower.

May help: breast pain, period pain, irregular periods, premenstrual syndrome, polycystic ovary syndrome, dry vagina and vulva, menopausal flushes, sweats, low libido

Part used: rootlets or rhizome

Actions: anti-inflammatory, diuretic, womb-stimulating, oestrogenic, hormone-balancing

Special notes: good for hormone imbalance associated with stress; useful when coming off HRT; tablets preferable, as tincture is so acrid

Caution: avoid if pregnant or breastfeeding (note the hormone-balancing and oestrogenic herb cautions above)

Burdock (*Arctium lappa*; beggar's buttons; gobo)

Plant with purple flowers and hooked bracts or 'burrs'.

May help: gynae cancers

Part used: whole plant

Actions: immunity-boosting, anti-infective, cancer-fighting

Special note: A traditional remedy for acne

Calendula (marigold, *Calendula officinalis*)

Plant with bright orange daisy-like flower.

May help: period pain, pelvic congestion

Part used: flowers

Actions: anti-inflammatory, anti-infective, astringent, anti-spasmodic

Caution: do not take internally if pregnant or breastfeeding

Catuaba (*Erythroxylum catuaba*; *Juniperus brasiliensis*)

Tree with yellow and orange flowers.

May help: low sex drive

Part used: bark

Actions: aphrodisiac (probably due to nerve stimulation)

Cramp bark (*Viburnum opulus*, guelder rose, snowball tree)

Bush with round clusters of white flowers.

May help: period pain

Part used: bark

Actions: astringent, antispasmodic

Special notes: bitter and can cause nausea, so best combined with cinnamon or ginger; also good for intestinal pain

Caution: buy a reputable brand, as other herbs, such as *Acer spicatum* (mountain maple), are often substituted for this; use in pregnancy to calm unwanted womb contractions only with supervision by a qualified herbalist

Cranesbill (*Geranium maculatum*, wild geranium, storksbilll)

Plant with pink or purple flower.

May help: heavy periods

Part used: whole plant

Actions: astringent

Special note: good for teenagers

Caution: do not self-prescribe as this herb is strong

Cypress (*Cupressus*)

Evergreen coniferous tree with scale-like leaves.

May help: menopausal flushes and sweats

Part used: cones

Actions: counteracts sensitivity of blood vessels

Dandelion (*Taraxacum officinale*)

Plant with yellow flowers.

May help: endometriosis

Part used: root, leaves

Actions: anti-inflammatory, diuretic, boosts oestrogen breakdown in the liver

Dong quai (*Angelica sinensis*, Chinese angelica, angelica root, *dong kwai, dang gai,* women's ginseng)

Graceful celery-scented plant with clusters of small white flowers.

May help: painful, heavy and irregular periods; premenstrual syndrome; endometriosis; low sex drive; menopausal flushes and sweats

Part used: root

Actions: anti-inflammatory, anti-infective, antispasmodic, womb tonic, possibly oestrogenic

Special notes: good for pelvic congestion; better with paeony than alone; regulates prostaglandin production

Caution: note the hormone-balancing and oestrogenic herb cautions above

Echinacea (*Echinacea angustifolia*, coneflower)

Plant with spiky, fragrant purple flower.

May help: pelvic inflammatory disease, candida, herpes, trichomonas

Part used: roots and rhizome

Actions: immunity-boosting, anti-infective

Caution: if you're due to have surgery, stop taking echinacea as early as possible before to prevent allergic reactions and immune suppression. Avoid if pregnant; take for no longer than two weeks as it becomes less effective after that

False unicorn root (*Chamaelirium luteum*, helonias root, starwort, blazing star root, devil's bit)

Plant with spikes of small greenish-white flower.

May help: breast lumpiness, heavy periods, irregular periods, premenstrual syndrome, endometriosis, fertility problems, polycystic ovary syndrome, fibroids

Part used: root and rhizome

Actions: womb tonic, oestrogenic, hormone-balancing

Special notes: helps regulate ovary function in the first half of the cycle; if tests show you aren't ovulating take it twice a day, perhaps with *Vitex*

Caution: note the hormone-balancing and oestrogenic herb cautions – and never self-prescribe as it can over-stimulate the ovaries above

Fennel (*Foeniculum vulgare*)

Yellow-flowered, liquorice-scented plant with feathery leaves.

May help: period pain, dry vagina and vulva

Part used: seeds

Actions: anti-inflammatory, slightly oestrogenic

Special note: may boost milk supply in breastfeeding women

Feverfew (*Tanacetum parthenium*)

Plant with little white yellow-centred flower.

May help: period pain, heavy periods, endometriosis

Part used: leaves

Actions: anti-inflammatory

Special notes: inhibits prostaglandin production; can eat the fresh leaves – in a Marmite sandwich, for example, to disguise the taste

Caution: avoid if pregnant or on blood-thinning drugs; prolonged use may cause mouth ulcers

Ginger (*Zingiber officinalis*)

Tall plant with small white flower.

May help: period pain, endometriosis, irritable bowel syndrome

Part used: rhizome

Actions: anti-inflammatory, anti-spasmodic

Special note: inhibits prostaglandin production

Ginseng (*Panax ginseng*, Chinese or Korean ginseng; Siberian ginseng is different = *Eleutherococcus senticosus*)

Small plant with bright red berries and 'humanoid' roots.

May help: heavy periods (probably because of prostaglandin inhibitors), low sex drive.

Part used: root

Actions: immunity-boosting, stimulating/relaxing, oestrogenic

Special notes: its oestrogenic effect may result from a direct action of its plant oestrogens or via effects on the hypothalamus and pituitary; boosts testosterone and sperm production in men; helps to lower high blood sugar

Caution: avoid if you have high blood pressure, acute asthma or an acute infection or if you drink a lot of coffee. It can cause irritability. Take only a short course and consult your doctor first if on blood-thinning drugs. Stop ginseng at least seven days before any surgery to prevent low blood sugar and bleeding

Goldenseal (*Hydrastis canadensis*, orange or yellow root)

Small plant with little white flowers and red berries.

May help: heavy periods, candida, trichomonas

Part used: rhizomes

Actions: anti-inflammatory, anti-infective, astringent, womb-relaxing

Caution: avoid if pregnant or breastfeeding, or with high blood pressure; take for no longer than three months

Greater periwinkle (*Vinca major*)

Plant with blue flower.

May help: heavy periods

Part used: aerial parts

Uses: astringent

Caution: do not self-prescribe as this herb is strong

Horsetail (*Equisetum arvense*)

Tall non-flowering plant with cone-like spore-producing stem tips.

May help: heavy periods, cystitis

Part used: aerial parts

Uses: anti-inflammatory, diuretic, astringent

Special note: probably contains prostaglandin inhibitors

Juniper (*Juniperus communis*)

Coniferous shrub or small tree with purple-green berry-like cones.

May help: bloating in premenstrual syndrome, cystitis

Part used: 'berries'

Uses: anti-inflammatory, anti-infective, diuretic

Special note: contains natural diuretics

Caution: safest taken under the supervision of a qualified herbalist; avoid if you are pregnant or have kidney disease

Lady's mantle (*Alchemilla vulgaris*, lion's foot)

Plant with small green flower.

May help: heavy periods, premenstrual syndrome, fibroids

Part used: aerial parts

Uses: anti-inflammatory, astringent

Caution: avoid if pregnant

Lemon balm (*Melissa officinalis*, bee balm, sweet balm)

Plant with white flower.

May help: period pain; melissa ointment helps herpes

Part used: aerial parts

Uses: anti-viral, antispasmodic

Liquorice (*Glycyrrhiza glabram*, licorice)

Small shrubby plant with small pink flower.

May help: acne and excess body hair, in polycystic ovary syndrome

Part used: root, underground stem

Uses: anti-inflammatory, anti-viral, diuretic, antispasmodic, stimulating or relaxing, oestrogenic

Special notes: helps to block conversion of testosterone to dihydrotestosterone; oversensitivity to this latter hormone encourages 'male-pattern' hair loss

Caution: note the hormone-balancing and oestrogenic herb cautions above; long-term use of high-dose liquorice can raise blood pressure and deplete potassium

Milk thistle (*Silybum marianum, marian thistle, liver herb, Carduus marianus*)

Tall plant with purple spiny flowerhead.

May help: hepatitis

Part used: seeds

Uses: counteracts liver infection, drugs and toxins

Motherwort (*Leonurus cardiaca, lion's tail, lion's ear*)

Plant with tiny pinkish-purple or white flower.

May help: period pain, premenstrual syndrome, menopausal flushes and sweats

Part used: aerial parts

Uses: antispasmodic, womb-stimulating or relaxing

Mugwort (*Artemisia vulgaris*)

Downy plant with spikes of yellowish or purple-brown flower.

May help: dull period pain, endometriosis, scanty periods

Part used: aerial parts

Uses: diuretic, womb stimulant

Caution: avoid if pregnant or breastfeeding

Muira puama (*Liriosma ovata*, potency wood)

Bush or small tree with small white jasmine-scented flowers.

May help: low sex drive

Part used: root

Uses: astringent, aphrodisiac (probably because it's a nerve stimulant)

Paeony (*Paeonia lactiflora,* white flowered = *bai shao*, red-flowered = *chi shao*)

Plant with white or red flowers.

May help: endometriosis, polycystic ovary syndrome

Part used: root

Uses: anti-inflammatory, antispasmodic, hormone-balancing

Caution: note the hormone-balancing and oestrogenic herb cautions above

Partridge berry (*Mitchella repens*; squaw berry, root or vine)

Small evergreen plant with white or pink flowers and red or white berries.

May help: heavy periods

Part used: aerial parts

Uses: diuretic, astringent, womb tonic

Caution: note the hormone-balancing and oestrogenic herb cautions above; don't confuse with either blue or black cohosh, each of which can be called squaw root.

Parsley (*Petroselinum crispum*)

Plant with finely cut leaves, insignificant greenish flowers, and a yellowish root.

May help: premenstrual syndrome

Part used: root, seeds

Uses: anti-inflammatory, diuretic, antispasmodic

Caution: avoid seeds and root if pregnant; don't take parsley seed tea for more than two weeks except under a qualified herbalist's supervision

Red clover (*Trifolium pratense*)

Small plant with pinkish-purple flower.

May help: breast pain, premenstrual syndrome

Part used: flowers

Uses: antispasmodic, oestrogenic

Special note: contains isoflavone plant oestrogens

Caution: note the hormone-balancing and oestrogenic herb cautions above

Sage (*Salvia officinalis*)

Silver-green-leaved aromatic plant.

May help: period pain, dry vagina and vulva, menopausal flushes and sweats

Part used: aerial parts

Uses: anti-inflammatory, immunity-boosting, anti-infective, astringent, antispasmodic, oestrogenic

Special note: contains plant oestrogens

Caution: avoid if pregnant or breastfeeding (discourages milk production); use for no longer than one week

Sarsarparilla (*Smilax aristolochiaefolia,* wild liquorice)

A climbing vine.

May help: polycystic ovary syndrome

Part used: root, rhizome

Uses: anti-inflammatory, anti-infective

Special note: seems to prevent testosterone from interacting with its cell receptors

Shepherd's purse (*Capsella bursa-pastoris*)

Plant with small white flowers and little heart-shaped pods.

May help: heavy periods

Part used: aerial parts

Uses: anti-inflammatory, anti-infective, diuretic, astringent

Special note: good for teenagers; a member of the cabbage family, and eaten as a food in Asia

Caution: avoid if you have an underactive thyroid

Skullcap (*Scutellaria lateriflora*)

Plant with small blue flower.

May help: premenstrual syndrome

Part used: aerial parts

Uses: anti-inflammatory, diuretic, astringent, relaxing, antispasmodic

St John's wort (*Hypericum perforatum*)

Plant with yellow flower.

May help: mild to moderate depression, for example, around the menopause

Part used: aerial parts

Uses: anti-inflammatory, astringent, anti-depressant

Caution: can make several drugs less effective, including anti-epilepsy drugs and the Pill, so consult your doctor first if you are on any other medication; stop taking at least five days before any surgery, to prevent it from diminishing the effects of certain drugs.

Uva ursi (*Arctostaphylos uva-ursi,* bearberry)

Low evergreen shrub with pink flowers and red berries.

May help: cystitis

Part used: aerial parts

Uses: anti-inflammatory, anti-infective, diuretic

Caution: avoid if pregnant

Vervain (*Verbena officinalis*)

Plant with tiny lilac flowers.

May help: period pain

Part used: aerial parts

Uses: astringent, relaxing, antispasmodic, promotes milk flow.

Caution: avoid if pregnant

***Vitex agnus castus* (*agnus castus*, chasteberry, chaste tree, monk's pepper)**

Tall shrub with palm-like leaflets, spikes of small, very fragrant, pale lavender flowers and peppercorn-sized seeds.

May help: breast lumpiness or pain; painful, heavy or irregular periods; premenstrual syndrome; endometriosis; fertility problems; polycystic ovary syndrome; fibroids; low sex drive; dry vagina and vulva; menopausal flushes and sweats

Part used: seeds

Uses: hormone-balancing

Special notes: can stimulate ovulation and increase luteinising hormone (and therefore progesterone) and prolactin (though can reduce follicle-stimulating hormone). Possibly acts via the hypothalamus. If hormone tests in the second half of the cycle reveal low progesterone (implying that you're not ovulating) consider taking Vitex *agnus castus* each morning, starting on the first day of a period. Has a dopamine-like action so can help to balance neurotransmitters. Can relieve bloating, fatigue, anxiety, and sugar craving. Stimulates milk production. Usually prescribed for three to nine months

Caution: note the hormone-balancing and oestrogenic herb cautions above; never self-prescribe for fertility problems

Wild yam (*Dioscorea villosa*, rheumatism or colic root)

Vine-like perennial with starchy, potato-like tubers.

May help: period pain, premenstrual syndrome, menopausal flushes and sweats

Part used: root, rhizome

Uses: anti-inflammatory, diuretic, antispasmodic, oestrogenic

Caution: note the hormone-balancing and oestrogenic herb cautions above

Yarrow (*Achillea millefolium*, nosebleed)

Plant with finely cut leaves and white or pink flowers.

May help: heavy periods

Part used: aerial parts

Uses: anti-inflammatory, anti-infective, astringent, womb tonic

Caution: avoid if pregnant

aromatherapy

Aromatherapy involves the use of oils extracted from plants – their 'essential oils'. Various combinations of naturally occurring chemicals in these oils can lift the spirits, relax, stimulate and aid healing.

Simply smelling an oil stimulates nerve endings in the nose, which sends messages to the brain. If you associate that scent with feeling relaxed, this encourages relaxation; if you associate it with feeling alert, it encourages alertness. Essential oils are useful for skin infections as they contain natural antiseptics and antibiotics. Some also contain plant hormones. Smaller molecules can influence health by passing through the lining of the breathing passages, or through the skin, into the bloodstream, where they are carried around the body. Good ways of inhaling a scent are by putting a few drops of oil into a little water that's then heated, or adding a few drops (mixed with some carrier oil to aid dispersion) to your bath water.

Aromatherapy massage

Try for: premenstrual syndrome, overweight and obesity.

Massage yourself – or have someone massage you – lubricating hands with some 'carrier' oil (see below) scented with one or more essential oils chosen for their particular properties. The possible healing effects include relaxation, relief from pain due to stress-induced muscle tension, and boosting of the circulation of blood and lymph. These effects occur not only in response to being touched, but also because of the oil's scent, and also – though this is much less important – because molecules from the oil are entering your body through your breathing passages and skin. Massage is also an excellent way for you to show concern and love for yourself, or for your masseur to show their concern and love for you.

Choose the carrier oil from sweet almond, apricot-kernel, grapeseed, jojoba, macadamia nut, peach kernel, wheatgerm or sunflower oils then add essential oils. Warm by standing the container in a bowl of hot water for five minutes.

Keep warm, and aim to do (or ask for) what feels best – there are no rules! One suggestion is to start by smoothing the affected part of your body gently with long strokes, then gradually try more vigorous movements (such as firmer stroking, kneading and patting) and finish with long, gentle, slow strokes again.

Aromatic abdominal compress

Try for: period pain, endometriosis, pelvic inflammatory disease, cystitis.

An aromatic compress can help reduce abdominal pain and muscle tension. Add one or two drops each of the required oils to a pint of hot water; immerse a flannel or small hand towel, then wring it out. Lie down, place the compress over your lower abdomen, cover with a dry towel and put a hot-water bottle on top. Now relax for at least half an hour.

Aromatic abdominal massage

Try for: period pain, cystitis, heavy, irregular, scanty or absent periods, endometriosis, premenstrual syndrome, irritable bowel syndrome, pelvic pain.

This is especially good for pain and stress.

Lubricate your skin with two teaspoons of sweet almond oil mixed with a total of six drops chosen from cypress, clary sage, geranium, lavender, Roman chamomile, or rose oils. Using the flat of one hand, gently massage your tummy, sweeping slowly around it with a smooth, slow, sweeping, continuous, clockwise stroke for several minutes.

Selected aromatherapy oils for gynae conditions

Besides choosing oils recommended for your disorder (see page 289), choose them also according to the scent that appeals the most. Many aromatherapists believe we are instinctively drawn to the oils that can do most good.

general cautions

- If you are pregnant, trying to get pregnant, or breastfeeding, use *only* lavender, citrus (neroli, bergamot, grapefuit, petitgrain, orange, lime), frankincense or ylang ylang oils.
- Avoid sunlight on skin to which you have recently applied citrus oil (though this is unnecessary after synthetic bergamot oil).
- Don't apply any essential oil other than tea tree and lavender directly to the skin – always add it to a carrier oil first.

The following oils are reputed to be:

Hormone-balancing – clary sage, geranium, rose, sweet fennel.

Diuretic – geranium, juniper, lavender, rosemary.

Stress-relieving – bergamot, chamomile, geranium, lavender, neroli, rose, ylang ylang.

Antiseptic – chamomile, geranium, juniper, lavender, marjoram, rosemary, tea tree.

Use the following oils for the gynae conditions listed:

Bergamot – premenstrual syndrome, any stress.

Chamomile – premenstrual syndrome any stress.

Clary sage – breast lumps; period pain; irregular, absent or scanty periods; premenstrual syndrome; menopausal flushes and sweats.

Cypress – painful or heavy periods.

Fennel – heavy, irregular, absent or scanty periods; menopausal flushes and sweats; overweight.

Frankincense – painful or heavy periods

Geranium – breast lumps; period pain; heavy, irregular, absent or scanty periods; premenstrual syndrome; dry vulva; menopausal flushes and sweats; overweight.

Ginger – low sex drive (note: do not add neat to bath water).

Grapefruit – overweight.

Juniper berry – painful, irregular, absent or scanty periods; vulva infection; cystitis; overweight.

Lavender – breast lumps, period pain, premenstrual syndrome, endometriosis, pelvic pain, herpes infection, menopausal flushes and sweats, cystitis, irritable bowel syndrome.

Lime – overweight.

Marjoram – painful, irregular, absent or scanty periods.

Neroli – premenstrual syndrome.

Rose – breast lumps; painful, heavy, irregular, absent or scanty periods; premenstrual syndrome; low sex drive; menopausal flushes and sweats.

Rosemary – period pain, heavy periods, premenstrual syndrome, overweight.

Sandalwood – low sex drive.

Tea tree – skin or vulva infections.

Ylang ylang – low sex drive, menopausal flushes and sweats.

light

Bright daylight

This helps to balance many hormones (including sex hormones) and neurotransmitters (including serotonin) and boosts our 'feel-good factor'.

May help: premenstrual syndrome, irregular periods, fertility problems, polycystic ovary syndrome, low sex drive, anxiety, gynae cancers, osteoporosis, overweight, bulimia, acne, fibromyalgia.

General advice regarding exposure to bright daylight:

•   Avoid sunburn when you expose your skin to bright outdoor daylight.

•   Older people may need more sunlight, and young babies shouldn't be exposed to direct sunlight.

•   If you can't go outside, sit by a window, since plain window glass transmits most light wavelengths well – although it cuts out some ultraviolet (UV) light (needed for vitamin D production), so open the window if you're warm enough.

•   If you wear glasses, spend a little time outdoors each day in bright daylight without them. This is because spectacle lenses filter out some UV light, yet it's possible that a little indirect UV in your eyes may have beneficial effects on your pineal gland and brain. (Note that too much UV damages the eyes.)

•   Avoid too much sunlight if you have premature skin ageing, skin cancer, cold sores, cataracts, age-related macular degeneration, rosacea, lupus or light-sensitive migraine. Avoid sunlight if you are on medication that sensitises you to light.

Bright light from a light box or visor

This can help to boost or rebalance various hormones and neurotransmitters and reset a disturbed body clock. It's especially useful for people who can't get enough bright daylight, or need extra helpings of bright light at particular times of day.

May help: premenstrual syndrome, irregular periods, polycystic ovary syndrome, fertility problems, low sex drive, anxiety, bulimia, gynae cancers, overweight, fibromyalgia.

Light box – The brighter the light, the faster its effects. Aim for one hour's daily exposure from a light box that produces 2,500 lux of light; 40 minutes if it produces 5,000 lux and 20 minutes if it produces 10,000 lux; more than two hours daily exposure may disturb sleep.

Light visor – this looks a little like a baseball cap and has battery-operated bright lights under its peak. Because the light source is so near the eyes, the light intensity producing beneficial effects is less than that needed from a light box. It may be possible to adjust it to 3,000 lux.

General advice

Check that the box or visor you buy is free from UV light and use it according to the manufacturer's instructions.

Flashing light mask

This can rebalance neurotransmitter levels, raise endorphin levels, speed slow brainwaves and help to reset a disturbed body clock.

May help: premenstrual syndrome, anxiety, overweight, migraine.

General advice

Close your eyes when wearing it. Start with a rate of 30 flashes a second, and if necessary, try adjusting it to between 8 and 50.

part four / what doctors can do

Some of the tests, investigations and treatments that were mentioned in Part Two and apply to several gynae disorders are discussed here in more detail, but if you need to know more you can ask your doctor, contact a relevant charity or self-help group or look on the Internet (see Helplist, page 313, for suggestions).

tests and investigations

Blood or saliva tests for hormone levels

For: breast swelling; irregular, scanty or absent periods, fertility problems, testing for fertility around the menopause.

What they involve: for a blood test a blood sample, usually from an arm vein, is sent to a laboratory for measurements of the levels of oestradiol (the 'strongest' oestrogen), progesterone, follicle stimulating hormone (FSH), luteinising hormone (LH) or testosterone. For a saliva test a sample of saliva is sent to a laboratory, again for hormone measurements. It's best to have several samples of blood or saliva taken at different times of the day, since hormone levels can fluctuate considerably.

sex hormone levels

There is a range of normal values for each hormone in different phases of the menstrual cycle (see also page 16).

	Follicular	Mid-cycle	Luteal
LH	1–12	16–79	1–10
FSH	3–12	8–20	1–9
Oestradiol	110–752	22–1,468	147–1,468
Progesterone			>30 = ovulatory cycle with adequate luteal phase
			NB: <10 = non-ovulatory cycle
			10–30 = ovulatory cycle with inadequate luteal phase

Testosterone 0.5–3

Postmenopausal levels

LH	14–77
FSH	35–150
Oestradiol	37–129

LH and FSH measurements are in international units per litre (iu/l; oestradiol in pico-moles per litre (pmol/l) and progesterone and testosterone in nano-moles per litre (nmol/l).

Special notes:

• Having a mid-cycle peak of FSH and LH shows that you are ovulating.

• Raised levels of FSH and LH in the second half of your cycle suggests that your ovaries aren't working properly.

• Low levels of FSH and LH in the second half of your cycle suggest that either your hypothalamus or pituitary is not working properly.

• A raised level of FSH can indicate a premature, early or normal menopause.

• A 'luteal defect' means that your corpus luteum isn't working properly (see page 21), or that it isn't there because you haven't ovulated. This can be demonstrated with a blood or saliva test for progesterone in the second half of your cycle. A blood test is most useful 7–9 days after ovulation (day 21 of your cycle, day 1 being the first day of your period). Low levels over several cycles suggest a luteal defect.

Swabs

For: nipple discharge; period pain; pelvic inflammatory disease; lump in vulva or vagina; sore, itchy vulva and/or vagina, perhaps with a discharge; dry vagina and vulva; bacterial vaginosis; candida; pelvic inflammatory disease; sexually transmitted infections.

What they involve: a doctor or nurse mops up a little moisture, discharge or cells from your nipple, vulva, vagina or cervix, usually using a sterile cotton bud. This 'swab' is sent to a laboratory for 'culture and sensitivity' tests which involve culturing (growing) any micro-organisms present in the swab, and applying several antibiotics to them to see which are most effective.

Ultrasound scan

For: breast lumps, period pain, heavy periods, fertility problems, ovary cyst, polycystic ovary syndrome, ovary cancer, fibroids, womb polyps, postmenopausal bleeding, pelvic pain.

What it involves: you will need a full bladder to get a good scan. A technician or doctor oils your skin, then slides the scanner over it to direct an ultrasound beam over the area. The scanner analyses its 'echo' to produce an on-screen image of the internal organs. Inserting the scanner in the vagina (for a 'transvaginal ultrasound scan') gives a clearer picture of the pelvic organs.

No discomfort is involved.

Mammogram

For: breast lumps or other changes, breast cancer.

What it involves: low-dose X-rays are done of each breast while it's compressed between metal 'plates'. Many women have some discomfort when their breast is compressed but it lasts only for a few seconds.

Special notes:

• A mammogram can identify small cancers several years before they can be felt.

• If you are premenopausal, a mammogram is most accurate in the two weeks before a period.

• If a mammogram suggests a lump, you may need another mammogram, then a needle biopsy.

• While some trials suggest that regular mammograms don't save lives, the general consensus is still that it's wise to have them.

Cervical smear (Papanicolou or 'Pap' smear)

For: ruling out pre-cancer or cancer; sore, itchy vulva and/or vagina, perhaps with a discharge; vulva cancer; postmenopausal bleeding.

What it involves: you lie on your back, knees bent, and a doctor or nurse inserts an instrument called a speculum into your vagina to open it and enable a view of your cervix. Next, they scrape some cells from the cervix, where the covering of its outer part meets the lining of its inner part. For a traditional 'dry' smear, cells are removed with a wooden spatula. (An 'extended-tip' spatula is twice as likely to collect enough cells as is the more usual broader-ended spatula.) The cells are smeared on a glass slide, sprayed with or dipped into 'fixing' liquid, then sent to the laboratory for examination. With a newer method ('liquid based cytology') cells are removed with a tiny brush that's rinsed or suspended in a special fluid. This is more likely to pick up enough cells, reducing the likelihood of needing a repeat smear.

Many women can sense when a smear is being taken but have no discomfort; a few notice slight soreness, and occasionally this persists for some days.

Special notes A smear is ideally done two weeks after the first day of your period.

An 'inadequate' smear means one of several things: too few cells, cells taken from the wrong place, cells have dried too soon, cells have been poorly preserved or not fixed well enough or blood or inflammatory cells are preventing a good view. In any of these situations the smear has to be done again.

Most women who have an 'abnormal' smear *do not* have cancer. However, abnormal cells become cancerous in some women, so your doctor will recommend a repeat smear, or a colposcopy (plus a biopsy if necessary).

Colposcopy

For: cervical erosion, abnormal smear, pelvic pain.

What it involves: you sit with your legs apart and feet up in rests, probably in a special 'colposcopy chair'. The doctor inserts an instrument called a speculum into your vagina to open it up. He or she then inserts a colposcope (like an illuminated telescope), looks closely at your cervix and takes a smear or biopsy or treats your cervix if necessary. You may see your cervix on a screen.

Possible complications from a biopsy or treatment include pain and bleeding, cervical infection and vaginal discharge. Avoid tampons and sex until these have cleared up.

Womb-lining (endometrial) biopsy

For: heavy periods, irregular periods, fertility problems, womb polyp, womb cancer, pelvic inflammatory disease, postmenopausal bleeding, bleeding after sex when a smear is normal.

What it involves: you lie on your back on a special bed with your feet up in stirrups, and a doctor inserts a speculum to open your vagina. He or she then inserts an instrument (such as a suction device

297

called a Pipelle aspirator that sucks out the womb lining or a curette, attached to a suction device, that cuts away the womb lining) and moves it around – which may be painful. A womb-lining biopsy can also be taken during hysteroscopy, perhaps with a transvaginal ultrasound scan to locate problem areas; another possibility, done under general anaesthetic, is a dilatation and curettage ('D and C') in which your cervix is opened and your womb lining scraped out.

Special notes: take a painkiller such as ibuprofen between thirty minutes and an hour before. A biopsy in the second half of the cycle can indicate whether your womb lining has thickened normally and ovulation is therefore likely to have occurred. A womb biopsy can miss small polyps or fibroids.

Possible complications include pain and bleeding for some days or weeks, womb infection or puncture and damage to the cervix.

Hysteroscopy

For: endometriosis in the womb, heavy periods, fertility problems, fibroids, womb polyps, womb cancer, pelvic inflammatory disease, postmenopausal bleeding.

What it involves: this may be done under general or local anaesthetic. A doctor passes an illuminated viewing tube via the vagina and through the cervix into the womb, to examine the inside of the womb. He or she can pass instruments up the tube and use them to take a womb-lining biopsy, for example, or remove small fibroids or polyps.

Special notes: one in four women has some pain afterwards; a little pain and bleeding may continue for a week to ten days or so after a biopsy.

A Pipelle biopsy (see above) can be more accurate.

Laparoscopy

For: sterilisation, endometriosis, fertility problems, ovary cysts, polycystic ovary syndrome, fibroids, ovary cancer, pelvic pain, pelvic inflammatory disease.

What it involves: this procedure is done under a general anaesthetic. The doctor passes a tube through a small incision in your umbilicus, and blows carbon dioxide gas around your organs for a better view. The tube is removed and a laparoscope (very fine illuminated viewing tube) passed through the incision. A tiny magnifier at the tip of the laparoscope is connected to a little camera that relays pictures to a screen. Other tiny incisions – usually in the 'bikini line' – enable 'keyhole' surgery, or treatment with, for example, an electrically heated wire loop or a laser beam.

You may need an overnight stay in hospital, and could have some abdominal pain and distension and, perhaps, temporary pain in your right shoulder due to trapped gas.

You should be able to resume everyday activities within a day or two, although more serious operations require longer recovery times.

Possible complications include perforation of the bowel or other organs.

prescribed drugs

Medical drugs are powerful and if carefully chosen can be very useful.

The following list contains brief details of most of the prescribed drugs mentioned in Part Two. Drugs used for only one gynae condition are described along with that condition in Part Two. It includes possible side effects (except for those of the Pill and HRT, which you'll find in Part One). Note that many side effects are extremely uncommon.

NSAIDs – non-steroidal anti-inflammatory drugs

(prescription-only NSAIDs include mefenamic acid, tranexamic acid, naproxen)

For: painful periods, heavy periods, endometriosis, fibroids.

How they work: reduce pain by inhibiting the production of inflammatory prostaglandins. The above NSAIDs are stronger than over-the-counter ones. Tranexamic acid reduces bleeding from the womb.

Special notes: some people are allergic to NSAIDs and should obviously avoid them. Avoid them too if you suffer from indigestion or peptic ulcer. Avoid alcohol as this can further irritate the stomach. Also avoid garlic, ginseng, ginkgo and vitamin E as these can thin the blood and encourage stomach bleeding.

Possible side effects include: nausea, diarrhoea, abdominal pain, dizziness, rash, headaches, vertigo, hearing disturbance, light sensitivity, blood in urine. More seriously, there may be stomach ulcers, mouth and throat swelling, breathing difficulty, kidney, liver, lung or pancreas damage.

Antibiotics

For: breast infections, inflamed Bartholin's gland, pelvic inflammatory disease, chlamydia infection, gonorrhoea, urine infection.

what to do when starting a drug

Your doctor will:

- check any 'contra-indications' (reasons why you shouldn't take it)
- consider whether any cautions over its use apply to you
- note any other prescribed or over-the-counter medications you are taking, and consider whether they could interact with the drug in question.

You should:

- ask your doctor or pharmacist about possible side effects and read any information that comes with the packaging
- contact your doctor or pharmacist if you develop an unacceptable side effect, are concerned about a side effect or have an unexpected reaction.

How they work: kill or disable bacteria.

Special notes: special cautions, interactions with other drugs and side effects vary with each antibiotic. Research suggests that while on antibiotics, it's worth taking a supplement of probiotics – 'good-guy' micro-organisms such as lactobacilli (from health stores, pharmacies and some supermarkets) – to help prevent diarrhoea.

Metronidazole

For: bacterial vaginosis, trichomonas.

How it works: antibiotic, and antiprotozoal (acts against one-celled organisms).

Special notes: avoid alcohol until 48 hours after completing the course, or it can cause severe nausea and vomiting, headache, abdominal pain, hot flushes, and palpitations.

Possible side effects include: nausea, vomiting, loss of appetite, abdominal pain, dark urine.

Antifungal drugs

For: candida, hepatitis.

How they work: kill infecting fungi.

Special notes: special cautions, interactions with other drugs and side effects vary with each drug.

Antiviral drugs

For: herpes infection, HIV.

How they work: prevent viruses from multiplying.

Special notes: special cautions, interactions with other drugs and side effects vary for each drug.

The Pill

Combined (oestrogen + progestogen) oral contraceptive Pill

(for side effects, see Part One, page 41)

For: contraception, painful or heavy periods; endometriosis; polycystic ovary syndrome; can also reduce a high risk of ovary cancer.

How it works: prevents ovulation and helps to correct hormone imbalance. The type, number and dose of oestrogens vary in different formulations, as do the type and dose of progestogen.

Special note: if you're on this Pill and have breast lumps and pain stopping it, or changing to a less oestrogenic one, may help.

Progestogens – including progestogen-only contraceptive Pill (for side effects see Part One, page 42)

For: contraception; painful, heavy or irregular periods; endometriosis; fibroids; pelvic pain.

How they work: prevent ovulation and reduce heavy bleeding.

Special note: thicken cervical mucus. Some progestogens, such as levonorgestrel, also have oestrogenic and androgenic actions.

Dose of oestrogen

If taking the combined Pill, it's wise to take one with a relatively low dose of oestrogen.

Risk factors to consider

Your doctor will ask about your risk factors and help you to weigh up the safety of the Pill for you as an individual.

Contraindications for taking the Pill, include:

- age over 50
- pregnancy
- breastfeeding a baby under six months old
- serious obesity – with a BMI (body mass index, see page 241) of 40 or more
- being bedridden
- history of certain types of migraine (such as attacks lasting over 72 hours despite treatment)
- smoking 40 or more cigarettes a day
- history of an abnormal internal blood clot (causing deep vein thrombosis, a stroke or a heart attack)
- blood pressure over 160/100
- leg in plaster
- diabetes complications
- unhealthy blood fats
- blood-clotting abnormality
- sclerosing treatment for varicose veins
- liver disease
- lupus
- breast, ovary or womb cancer
- family history of breast cancer
- unexplained vaginal bleeding
- certain risk factors – see below – for a blood clot in the leg (deep vein thrombosis), stroke or heart attack.

Risk factors for blood clots

Many factors encourage blood clots (see HRT, page 306, for a full list), but those listed here are particularly important à propos the Pill.

The Pill could be suitable if you have just one of these risk factors but should be avoided if you have two or more:

- family history, with your mother or sister having had a clot in a leg vein under the age of 45. (Note: all women with this family history should avoid Pills containing the progestogens desogestrel or gestodene)
- moderate obesity – a body mass index of 30-40
- long-term immobilisation – e.g. in a wheelchair
- varicose veins

Risk factors for heart attacks and strokes

Many factors encourage heart attacks and strokes (see HRT, page 306, for a full list), but those listed here are particularly relevant to women taking the Pill.

The Pill could be suitable if you have just one of these risk factors, but should be avoided if you have two or more:

- age over 35
- family history of arterial disease (such as heart attacks or strokes) in close relative, such as a parent or sibling
- diabetes
- high blood pressure
- obesity
- smoker
- migraine

Looking after yourself on the Pill

- Before prescribing the Pill your doctor will examine you and ask questions about your personal and family health history so as to reduce the risk of certain side effects

- Take the Pill at around the same time each day. If you're more than 12 hours late you may not be protected against getting pregnant

- Contact your doctor if you develop any side effects

- Get urgent medical help if you develop unexplained pain in a calf, chest pain or shortness of breath

- If you are a migraineur (migraine sufferer) report any increase in the frequency of your headaches and get urgent medical help for atypical migraine symptoms lasting more than one hour

- Note that the Pill provides no protection against catching or spreading sexually transmitted infections

- Have an annual blood-pressure check

Progestogen-releasing intra-uterine system (see Part One, page 43).

For: contraception, heavy periods, endometriosis, fibroids.

How it works: prevents ovulation and reduces heavy bleeding.

Gonadotrophin-release inhibitors (danazol, gestrinone)

For: breast lumps, breast pain, endometriosis.

How they work: act as anti-oestrogens by inhibiting the mid-cycle rise in gonadotrophins (follicle stimulating hormone and luteinising hormone); also have androgenic action.

Special notes: can raise sex drive. Their side effects are unacceptable to some women.

Possible side effects include: androgenic symptoms (weight gain, greasy skin, excess body hair and/or acne – in one in three women); nausea, dizziness, rash, backache, jaundice, period disturbances, menopausal symptoms (hot flushes, dry vagina, smaller breasts, poor sleep, weight gain, fluid retention, cramp, depression, osteoporosis). Gestrinone carries a higher risk of androgenic side effects, danazol of cramps and weight gain. These drugs have a weaker anti-oestrogen action than that of GnRH (see below), so less likely to cause hot flushes.

Gonadotrophin-releasing hormone (GnRH – or gonadorelin) analogues (synthetic 'look-alike' drugs) (such as buserelin, goserelin, leuprorelin, nafarelin, triptorelin)

For: breast lumps, endometriosis, infertility, anaemia due to fibroids, for shrinking fibroids or the womb lining before womb surgery, premature puberty, pelvic pain.

How they work: they lower the oestrogen level. As they are much more active than human GnRH, they initially produce unnaturally high levels of luteinising hormone (LH) and follicle stimulating hormone (FSH). This stimulates the ovaries to produce so much oestrogen that it 'down-regulates' pituitary GnRH receptors, reducing FSH and LH production over two to four weeks. This reduces ovary stimulation and oestrogen production.

Special notes: their side effects can be unacceptable

Possible side effects include: reversible menopausal symptoms and signs that can be prevented with HRT.

Bromocriptine

For: breast lumps; breast pain, fertility problems.

How it works: reduces a raised prolactin level.

Special notes: avoid alcohol. Use non-hormonal contraception as bromocriptine may trigger ovulation.

Possible side effects include: nausea; faintness; dizziness; headache;vomiting; constipation; numb, white fingers; confusion; drowsiness; hallucinations; abnormal movements; dry mouth; leg cramps.

Clomiphene

For: irregular periods, fertility problems, polycystic ovary syndrome.

How it works: can stimulate ovulation by blocking oestrogen cell receptors, so stimulating increased production of follicle stimulating hormone (FSH) and luteinising hormone (LH). Start on fifth day of period and take for five consecutive days in each of three cycles.

Special notes: there is a suspicion that it encourages breast or ovary cancer later. Report any side effects to your doctor.

Possible side effects include: hot flushes, abdominal pain, rash, hair thinning, visual disturbance, ovarian hyperstimulation syndrome (enlarged ovaries, and excess fluid between the abdominal wall and abdominal organs and around the lungs and heart).

HRT (hormone replacement therapy)

For: heavy periods near menopause; menopausal flushes, sweats and, perhaps, low libido, poor memory and 'cystitis'; osteoporosis (prevention or treatment); prolapse; dry vagina and vulva; itchy vulva and/or vagina and, perhaps, discharge; menopausal symptoms from danazol, gestrinone, or gonadotrophin-releasing hormone therapy (see above).

How it works: raises the body's oestrogen level.

Possible side effects: see Part One, page 36.

Special notes: Some women stay on HRT for many months or years, so it's important to be well aware of the choices and possible side effects.

Formulations

There are many formulations to suit different needs; they provide oestrogen plus progestogen ('combined HRT'); oestrogen alone; progestogens or progesterone alone; or there is a drug called tibolone that has a combination of oestrogenic, progestogenic and androgenic actions.

Oestrogen helps to prevent menopause-related symptoms triggered by a woman's own oestrogen falling, fluctuating or being low.

HRT contains either mixed ('conjugated') oestrogens from mares' urine, or oestrogen (usually oestradiol) made in the laboratory from yams, soy beans or other plants.

Possible progestogens include norethisterone, levonorgestrel, medroxyprogesterone acetate, norgestrel and dydrogesterone. Progesterone is available too.

Combined HRT – This is for women who still have their womb and it's what most women who take HRT start on. Besides containing one or more oestrogens, it also contains a progestogen, since while oestrogen encourages womb cancer, progestogens discourage it.

Women on oestrogen who need progestogen but don't want the possible side effects of progestogens from tablets or patches can use a progesterone-only vaginal gel, since enough progesterone reaches the womb to cause periods (and so prevent potentially risky thickening of the womb lining) but there isn't enough in the blood to cause side effects such as headaches and bloating. There has been a lot of interest in progesterone cream, but a recent study showed that the amount of progesterone absorbed from the skin into the blood isn't enough to protect the womb lining.

Periods or bleed-free?

• 'Sequential combined' HRT. Besides oestrogen each day, this provides progestogen for 10-14 days every

month or three months, causing monthly or quarterly periods.

• 'Continuous combined' HRT. This provides the same amounts of oestrogen and progestogen (or of tibolone) each day, so a woman has no periods (though it may take some months to become bleed-free and a very few women never do). It's suitable if you still have your womb and your last 'natural' period was more than 12 months ago, if you've been on sequential combined HRT for over five years or if you're aged 55 or over.

Oestrogen-only HRT – 'Whole-body' oestrogen-only HRT (HRT that enters the bloodstream and affects the whole body, such as from tablets or patches) is only for women who've had a hysterectomy.

If you still have your womb, you can use an oestrogen-only vaginal cream, pessary or ring for three months without taking progestogens, since so little oestrogen applied this way gets into the bloodstream and reaches the womb, where it would thicken the womb lining. However, if you use an oestrogen vaginal cream, pessary or ring regularly, for more than three months, it's wise to take progestogen tablets or patches or use a progesterone vaginal gel, to counteract oestrogen's potentially risky womb-thickening effect.

Dose of oestrogen in HRT

Take a preparation that provides the lowest dose of oestrogen that relieves your symptoms. Lower-dose (lower-oestrogen) HRT is available as tablets providing 1mg of oestradiol or 0.625mg of conjugated oestrogens a day and patches providing 25-50 mcg of oestradiol a day. Adjust the dose of gel, cream or nasal spray by using more or less of the product. A lower dose of oestrogen is as effective as a higher dose for hot flushes.

How to take it – HRT that affects the whole body is available as tablets, skin patches (worn on the lower back or upper thigh), tablets plus patches, skin gel, nasal spray and implants (oestrogen pellets inserted under the skin).

Oestrogen-only vaginal creams, gels or pessaries are available for vagina, vulva or bladder problems.

Making the decision

Each woman needs to weigh up – perhaps with her doctor's help – the benefits and risks for herself as an individual.

For example:

- If considering short-term HRT for flushes and sweats, you might not worry too much about it increasing the risk of breast cancer unless your risk of this is high. This is because the increased risk of breast cancer from HRT is very small in the first five years, and you won't stay on it any longer.

- If considering long-term HRT to reduce a raised risk of osteoporosis and if you also have a raised risk of breast cancer or heart disease, discuss with your doctor whether it's advisable for you to take a bone-protecting drug called a SERM (selective oestrogen receptor modulator, such as raloxifene) instead.

- If you've been taking higher-dose HRT to control flushes and sweats because a lower-dose product didn't help and you want to stay on it long term for whatever reason, consider switching to lower-dose HRT after five years.

Risk factors to consider

HRT is unsuitable if you have an undiagnosed breast lump or postmenopausal bleeding; if you could be pregnant or if you have a history of severe liver disease, womb cancer or oestrogen-sensitive breast cancer.

HRT is one of many risk factors for breast cancer, heart attacks, strokes and blood clots, which puts some women off it. However, others prefer to assess their overall risk. Having several other risk factors for any one condition may make them decide not to add to their overall risk by taking HRT. But having few or no other risk factors might encourage them to accept the (relatively small) risk from HRT. In general, the more risk factors you have, the higher is your overall risk for that condition, though some factors (such as age for breast cancer) are more significant than others. You may want to consider HRT if you have a raised risk of osteoporosis (see page 232).

Does HRT make you gain weight?

Overall, studies show that women on HRT are no more likely to pile on the pounds than are other women. If we gain weight in our 50s and 60s it's generally because we have slowed down and take less exercise. However, HRT can encourage weight gain

other healthy-diet tips

Use these lists to note your risk factors before discussing your situation with your doctor:

Risk factors for breast cancer

- age (your risk rises each year)
- living in a developed country
- history of breast lumps
- started periods very young, had no children, had first child in your 30s, didn't breastfeed or had menopause over 55
- family history of breast, ovary or colon cancer
- too little exposure to bright outdoor daylight
- overweight
- unhealthy diet
- drink more than one alcohol unit a day (see page 75)
- history of heavy periods
- on the Pill some time in last 10 years
- physical inactivity
- smoking or passive smoking
- years of repeated use of dark brown or black hair dye (see page 76)
- HRT

Risk factors for blood clots

- being aged over 40
- overweight
- physical inactivity
- smoking
- inflamed veins (phlebitis)
- cancer
- previous blood clot
- recent injury or operation
- lupus (in which inflamed arteries cause a wide variety of symptoms)
- a flight longer than two hours, or other lengthy seated travel
- HRT

Risk factors for heart attacks and strokes

- age
- overweight (especially with much fat around waist)
- diabetes (type 2, the sort that tends to come on in later life)
- smoking
- unhealthy diet
- high blood pressure
- family history of arterial disease
- lack of exercise
- high total cholesterol, LDL-cholesterol, and triglyceride fats, and low HDL-cholesterol
- stress (especially if there is little control over stress and lack of support)
- emotional problems (researchers have specifically highlighted loneliness, heartbreak, hostility, anger and a lack of joy)
- going out poorly protected against cold weather
- commonly breathing air polluted with vehicle-exhaust fumes
- metabolic syndrome ('syndrome X') – the combination of obesity, high blood pressure, high insulin and blood-fat levels, a low HDL-cholesterol level and 'sticky' blood that clots easily
- underactive thyroid
- continued infection (e.g. peptic ulcer)
- possibly HRT

by making you retain fluid. Suspect this if you are bloated and have tight rings, or indentations in your skin from underwear and night-clothes.

Looking after yourself on HRT

- Before starting HRT, your doctor will check your blood pressure, height and weight. Some doctors do a pelvic examination and cervical smear. An ultrasound scan to assess the size of your ovaries and the thickness of your womb lining may be advisable if you have a history of period problems and/or fibroids.

- See your doctor every three months until free from troublesome menopausal symptoms or HRT-side-effects; then have routine checks as recommended. Note that HRT may take months to control menopausal symptoms.

- Report any side effects to your doctor (for example, if you develop migraine for the first time) as a different product may suit you better. For example, a smaller dose of oestrogen might be preferable if you retain fluid; patches, gel or spray if you have nausea, bloating or cramps; and a different progestogen – or vaginal progesterone – if you have depression or acne.

- Get urgent medical help if you develop unexplained pain in your calf, chest pain or shortness of breath.

- If you are on long-term HRT, your doctor will probably recommend a smaller dose of oestrogen as you get older. Recent research found low-dose HRT as successful as high-dose HRT at preventing osteoporosis.

- Be 'breast-aware', quickly report anything unexpected and go for regular mammograms. If you develop breast lumps or breast pain, stopping HRT or switching to a less oestrogenic formulation may help.

- If you have risk factors other than HRT for blood clots and you're going to be travelling seated (for example, in a plane, train, car or coach) for more than two hours, tell your doctor well before you go. This is because you may benefit from temporary precautions (such as wearing elastic stockings or taking blood-thinning medication) to help prevent a blood clot.

- Tell your doctor if you become immobilised.

- Don't use an HRT pessary or cream before sex, or your partner could absorb the hormones.

- Every year, revisit the lists of risk factors above and weigh up afresh the pros and cons of continuing HRT.

- **Note :** HRT does not provide contraception! Remember that you are potentially fertile for two years after you have had your last period if this was before you were 50, and for one year if you were over 50.

How long to stay on HRT

- If you take HRT for menopausal symptoms your doctor may advise continuing for two to five years, after which they are unlikely to recur.

- If you're on long-term HRT to reduce a high risk of osteoporosis, note that its protection lasts only for as long as you are taking it. Some experts suggest switching to other bone-protective drugs as you near the age of 60.

- You and your doctor may think it wise for you to avoid long-term HRT if you have a high risk of breast cancer, heart disease or blood clots.

- If you develop breast or womb cancer while on HRT you may be interested to know that the life expectancy of women who opt to continue HRT after treatment for breast or womb cancer is no less than that of those who stop HRT.

Note : one in three women on HRT gives up, half within a year, because of side effects or concern that they might occur. Whenever you stop, reduce your dose gradually over two to three months to help prevent flushes and sweats from returning.

Tamoxifen

For: breast cancer (or if you are at a high risk); fertility problems.

How it works: latches on to oestrogen receptors on cells, where it can act as an oestrogen and stimulate gonadotrophin production. In certain other cells, though, it blocks a woman's own oestrogen, meaning it acts as an 'anti-oestrogen'. (Unfortunately, it acts as an oestrogen in the womb, meaning it stimulates womb cells and may encourage womb cancer. This can be watched for so as to facilitate early treatment, meaning that the benefits of tamoxifen, in terms of saving lives from breast cancer, far outweigh the increased risk of dying from womb cancer).

Special notes: report abnormal vaginal bleeding or discharge to your doctor.

Possible side effects include: stops periods in up to 71 per cent of women; can cause hot flushes, vaginal bleeding, vaginal discharge, nausea, headache, eye changes, rash, premature ovarian failure and, rarely, hypersensitivity, lung inflammation, blood clots, womb cancer.

Chemotherapy

For: any cancer.

How it works: destroys any rapidly dividing cells, including some healthy ones and cancer cells.

Special notes: can damage hair follicle cells, stomach and gut lining cells, immune system cells and bone marrow cells.

Can also damage ovaries and cause infertility. This happens, for example, in around three in every four women who have chemotherapy for breast cancer. However, animal research suggests that in as little as five years from now, a woman may be able to have an ovary removed and frozen before starting chemotherapy. If her cancer is cured and she wants a child, reinserting the ovary into her body might result in the possibility of pregnancy.

Possible side effects include: hair loss, poor resistance to infection, anaemia, bruising, bleeding, nausea, vomiting, diarrhoea, mouth ulcers, infertility.

surgery

An operation is an excellent treatment for certain conditions, although it should be done as a last resort if there are satisfactory non-surgical options.

Bear in mind that every operation can have complications. These can occur during surgery (for example, bleeding or an adverse reaction to the anaesthetic) or afterwards (for example, bleeding or wound infection). Also, pain and tenderness around the operation site are normal for some time afterwards.

Any operation used for only one gynae condition – such as mastectomy for breast cancer – is explained in Part Two.

Endometrial resection or ablation

(removal or destruction of the womb lining; 'TCRE' = transcervical resection of the endometrium)

For: heavy periods, small fibroids.

How it's done: You'll have a general anaesthetic. A doctor may do a resection by looking into the womb through a hysteroscope, distending and irrigating the womb with a special liquid and destroying part of the womb lining with heat from an electrically heated wire loop or a 'rollerball', or a laser beam. Newer methods, without a hysteroscope, mostly involve using heat (for example, from microwaves, radio-frequency waves, a laser beam or electrical energy), though one involves freezing.

Special notes: destroys up to 6mm ($^1/_4$in) depth of womb lining. Most likely to be effective just after a period when the womb lining is at its thinnest and least

after a gynae operation

Your health-care professionals will give you personal advice. The following are more general guidelines however. Use only pads (not tampons) after surgery involving the vagina or done via the vagina.

• Tell your doctor about any severe pain, or bright red, heavy or clotted vaginal bleeding after surgery.

• Don't drive or do anything requiring skill or concentration for 48 hours after a general anaesthetic.

• Avoid sexual activity until your doctor gives you the all clear (usually around six weeks), or at least until you no longer have a vaginal discharge; sexual arousal could stretch the vagina and delay healing.

• When you return to sex you may need a lubricant such as saliva or K-Y jelly.

• It's wise to do pelvic floor exercises from the first day after any gynae surgery and, after abdominal surgery, to ask a physiotherapist about exercises to strengthen your abdominal muscles.

likely to bleed or after the womb lining has been thinned by taking drugs (such as the GnRH analogue leuprorelin) for three months – though you may not like the side effects.

Afterwards periods stop in 30-50 per cent of women and are lighter in 35-65 per cent. But one in four women has recurrent problems and needs another endometrial resection or a hysterectomy. Not suitable if you might want to get pregnant in the future. Its long-term success is still being evaluated.

Possible complications: period-type pains, bleeding, a brownish discharge (for up to six weeks), urine infection, fluid overload from the absorption of irrigating liquid into the bloodstream, perforation of the womb plus damage of the bowel or bladder. The latter occurs in one in 130 women treated with a wire loop or microwaves and necessitates a hysterectomy.

Hysterectomy

For: heavy or irregular periods; endometriosis; fibroids; prolapse; cervix, womb, ovary or vagina cancer.

How it's done: under general anaesthetic. May be 'total' (including removal of the cervix); sub-total (leaving the cervix); or, for cancer, extended or 'radical' (including ovaries, upper vagina and, perhaps, lymph nodes). A total hysterectomy can be done via the vagina or via the abdomen through one largish cut, usually in the bikini line or as a 'keyhole' operation. Keyhole surgery involves several small incisions and is done with the surgeon looking through a laparoscope fitted with a miniature video camera that relays pictures of the inside of the abdomen and pelvis to a screen. Sub-total hysterectomies are always done through the abdomen. Having one of these may mean sex is more pleasurable than after a total one but there is a continuing possibility of cervix cancer, so you still need regular smears.

Recovery: Return to driving when you can reliably put both feet down for an emergency stop, probably after about four weeks. Gentle penetrative sex may be possible after about six weeks but check with your gynaecologist. Avoid heavy lifting for at least six to eight weeks. You'll probably be off work for at least six weeks, possibly several months.

Special notes: Hysterectomy should be a last resort for heavy periods, endometriosis or fibroids but many women in countries such as the US, UK and Brazil have it done before trying all the non-surgical options. Despite the fact that many women are pleased to be symptom-free this is unwise in view of the possible complications (see below). If a gynaecologist recommends a hysterectomy but you are unsure, get a second opinion.

If you have a hysterectomy before your menopause your ovaries are likely to fail – meaning that they no longer enable cyclical menstrual hormone swings or ovulation – earlier than they would otherwise have done. In up to one woman in three the ovaries fail within five years. Unless you get hot flushes, night sweats and, perhaps, other menopausal signs, you won't know this has happened because after a hysterectomy you no longer have periods to indicate that your ovaries are still active. So, if you have a hysterectomy in your 20s, 30s or 40s and before the menopause, it's wise to have tests for luteinising hormone (LH) and follicle stimulating hormone (FSH) every two or three years to see if you are still ovulating. This way, if you are relatively young, you can consider starting HRT as soon as your ovaries start to fail, so as to reduce the raised risk of osteoporosis that follows ovarian failure.

If you are postmenopausal the surgeon will probably recommend removing your ovaries too, to prevent future ovary disease. Surgeons may also recommend this for a young premenopausal woman, claiming she can take HRT to replace her ovarian hormones. However, removing the ovaries is more acceptable if a woman has a raised risk of ovary cancer.

Possible complications: occur in up to 45 per cent and include pain, bleeding, wound infection, urine infection and, in one in 2,000 healthy women, death – caused, for example, by massive and uncontrollable bleeding on the operating table or by a pulmonary embolism (a blood clot in a lung) occurring within a short time – usually a few weeks – of the operation. A hysterectomy increases the risk of developing incontinence in later life

by 60 per cent. Some women say sex is better afterwards, some that it's less pleasurable. Straightforward abdominal hysterectomy is most common and least likely to cause complications. However, laparoscopic-assisted abdominal hysterectomy has the highest complication rate. After hysterectomy some women find themselves grieving the loss of their ability to bear children.

Oophorectomy (removal of one or both ovaries)

For: severe endometriosis, ovary cyst, ovary cancer, high risk of breast or ovary cancer.

How it's done: under general anaesthetic. The surgeon removes one or both ovaries either via an incision made low in your abdomen or via a laparoscope.

Recovery: you may have some abdominal pain. You'll be able to return to most activities within two to four weeks.

Special notes: if you have ovary cancer your womb and cervix may also be removed. If you were premenopausal before having both ovaries removed you will have now have an unnaturally early menopause, so HRT may be beneficial, especially if you are relatively young, to reduce the raised risk of osteoporosis.

Possible complications: infection, adhesions (potentially hazardous strands of internal scar tissue, see page 184), bowel or bladder damage.

radiotherapy

May help: cancer.

What it is: ionising radiation destroys cells that are dividing very rapidly, or prevents them from multiplying.

How it's done: radiotherapists calculate very carefully the dose of radiation needed, so it's as low as possible, and the risk of complications minimised. A course of radiotherapy generally takes place over several weeks.

Special notes: a small trial suggests that 25 minutes of radiotherapy from a device placed in the open breast immediately after removal of a cancerous lump, helps to kill any remaining cancer cells and obviates the need for six weeks of daily radiotherapy. A larger trial is under way.

Possible side effects and complications: diarrhoea, abdominal cramps, cystitis, increased risk of incontinence in later life (although this risk is very much smaller than it used to be).

helplist

Most of the contacts in this list are based in the UK, but all websites should direct you to relevant worldwide links. If telephoning from outside the UK, use your country's code for 'international' followed by 44 (the national code for the UK), then the number given minus its first zero. For example, to reach Action for ME, the first contact given below, dial international + 44 1749 670799

Health-care charities and other organisations

Action for ME
PO Box 1302, Wells, Somerset BA5 1YE; tel. 01749 670799; www.afme.org.uk

Breast Cancer Care
Kiln House, 210 New King's Road, London SW6 4NZ; tel. 020 7384 or 020 7384 2984; www.breastcancercare.org.uk

Breast Cancer Network Australia
PO Box 4082, Auburn South Vic 3122; tel. 0061 3 9805 2500; www.bcna.org.au

Bristol Cancer Help Centre
Grove House, Cornwallis Grove, Clifton, Bristol BS8 4PG; tel. 0117 980 9500 or helpline 0117 980 9505

Canadian Breast Cancer Foundation
A charity involved with research, education and treatment; www.cbcf.org

Canadian Women's Health Network
A network of individuals, groups, organisations and institutions concerned with women's health; www.cwhn.ca/about/html

Cancer BACUP
3 Bath Place, Rivington Street, London EC2A 3JR; tel. 020 7920 7220 or 020 7696 9003; www.cancerbacup.org.uk

Cancer Research UK
61 Lincoln's Inn Fields, London WC2A 3PX; tel. 020 7061 8355; www.cancerresearchuk.org; information service www.cancerhelp.org.uk

Coeliac UK
PO Box 220, High Wycombe, Bucks HP11 2HY; tel. 01494 437278; UK helpline 0870 444 8804

Continence Foundation
307 Hatton Square, 16 Baldwins Gardens, London EC1N 7RT; tel. 020 7404 6875; UK helpline 0845 345 0165

Daisy Network *(for women who have an early menopause)*
PO Box 392, High Wycombe, Bucks HP15 7SH (send a sae); www.daisynetwork.org.uk

Family Planning Association
27-35 Mortimer Street, London W1N 7RJ; tel. 020 7636 7866; www.fpa.org.uk

Foresight *(Association for the Promotion of Preconceptual Care)*
Large sae to 28 The Paddock, Godalming, Surrey GU7 1XD; tel. 01483 427839; www.foresight-preconception.org.uk

Herpes Viruses Association
41 North Road, London N7 9DP; tel. 020 7609 9067; www.herpes.org.uk

International Union Against Cancer
Lists voluntary organisations; www.uicc.org/public/directory

International Cancer Information Services
Lists organisations around the world; www.cis.nci.nih.gov/resources/intlist.htm

Interstitial Cystitis Support Group
76 High Street, Stony Stratford, Buckinghamshire MK11 1AH; www.interstitialcystitis.co.uk

Lymphoedema Support Network
St Luke's Crypt, Sydney Street, London SW3 6NH; tel. 020 7351 4480; www.lymphoedema.org/lsn

National Association for Premenstrual Syndrome
41, Old Road, East Peckham, Kent TN12 5AP; tel. 0870 777 2177; www.pms.org.uk

National Endometriosis Society
50 Westminster Palace Gardens, 127 Artillery Row, London SW1P 1RL; tel. 020 7222 2781 or freephone 0808 808 2227; www.endo.org.uk

National Institute of Medical Herbalists
56 Longbrook Street, Exeter, Devon EX4 6AH; tel. 01392 426022; for a list of UK herbalists, send large sae.

National Lichen Sclerosus Support Group
PO Box 7600, Hungerford, RG17 7XD (send an sae); www.lichensclerosus.org

National Osteoporosis Society
Camerton, Bath BA2 0PJ; tel. 01761 471771 or helpline 01761 472721; www.nos.org.uk

Obgyn.net
A site providing information about gynaecology and a forum for discussion.

Ovacome
(For ovary cancer); St. Bartholomew's Hospital, West Smithfield, London EC1A 7BE; tel. 020 7600 5141; www.ovacome.org.uk

Polycystic Ovarian Syndrome Association
PO Box 80517, Portland, Oregon 97280; tel. (001) 877-775-PCOS; www.pcossupport.org

Quitline
(for stop-smoking help in the UK) tel. 0800 00 22 00

SHE (Simply Holistic Endometriosis) Trust
Red Hall Lodge Offices, Red Hall Drive, Bracebridge Heath, Lincoln LN4 2JT; tel. 01522 519992; www.shetrust.org.uk

Sjögren's Syndrome Foundation
www.sjogrens.com

US National Cancer Institute
tel.(00)1-800-4-CANCER; www.cancer.gov/cancer_information

Verity *(polycystic ovaries self-help group)*
52-54 Featherstone Street, London EC1Y 8RT; www.verity.pcos.org.uk

Wellbeing *(health research charity for women and babies)*
27 Sussex Place, Regent's Park, London NW1 4SP; tel. 020 7772 6400; www.wellbeing.org.uk

Other services or information

Breast Implants
(information for women considering implants)
Free (to UK) from Department of Health, PO Box 777, London SE1 6XH, quoting reference number 21218 1P 80k Sept 00 (CWP); or at www.doh.gov.uk/bimplant

Cancer treatment trials
Details of UK trials; www.cancerhelp.org.uk

Conticare catalogue
(continence products)
Shiloh Health Care Limited, Park Mill, Royton, Oldham OL2 6PZ; tel. 0800 917 0625

Medical information search
Information, for a fee, on books, leaflets, support groups and contacts, articles and research reports.
Meducation Ltd, 156 Middlewich Road, Sandbach, Cheshire CW11 1FH, UK; tel. 07818 428581; www.meducationltd.co.uk

Menopause Exchange,
PO Box 205, Bushey, Herts WD23 1ZS; tel. 020 8420 7245

Toxic Shock Syndrome Information Service
(funded by tampon manufacturers) PO Box 450, Godalming, Surrey GU7 1GR; tel. 020 7617 8040; www.tssis.com

Health-care products

Chlamydia test kit

This involves sending urine, collectedin the little pot, provided with the kit, to a lab and having the results returned to you by post;
The WB013 Chlamydia Home Test Kit costs £43.95; www.self-test-kits.co.uk

Contiform (*plastic tampon-like device*)
0044 1293 606 741

Head cooling during chemotherapy (*to help prevent hair loss*)
Hospital head cooling systems:
MSC, 274 Hither Green Lane, London SE13 6TT; tel. 020 8244 4040

Paxman Coolers Limited; tel. 01484 349 444; www.paxman-coolers.co.uk

Intermark Medical Innovations Ltd, tel. 020 8467 3355; www.intermarkmedical.com

Or buy a cool cap (CoolCap, from UK pharmacies, quoting PIP Code 2618247, or ScanMed International Ltd – in the UK: 0800 074 4469), and take it to hospital ready cooled in a freezer bag. This isn't as cold as a hospital cap, but may help.

Electronic ovulation monitor
The Persona Monitor, plus batteries and two months of urine-testing sticks, costs £64.95 and is available from leading pharmacies

Flor-Essence
Revital tel 0800 252875 (UK only)

Herbal remedies
Potter's (Herbal Supplies) Limited, Leyland Mill Lane, Wigan, Lancashire WN1 2SB; tel. 01942 405 100; www.herbal-direct.com

Napiers Herbalists; tel. 0131 343 6683; www.napier.net

Holland and Barrett
Food supplements, herbal remedies, essential oils, etc,
tel. 0870 606 6605; www.hollandandbarrett.com

Light boxes (*produce bright light of up to 10,000 lux*) and visors (*produce bright light up to 3,000 lux*)

Outside In (Cambridge) Ltd, 21 Scotland Road Estate, Dry Drayton, Cambridge CB3 8AT; tel. 01954 211 955; www.outsidein.co.uk

SAD Lightbox Co Ltd, Unit 48, Marlow Road, Stokenchurch, High Wycombe HP14 3QT; tel. 01494 448727; www.sad.uk.com

Bio-Brite Inc, 4350 East West Highway, Suite 401W, Bethesda, MD 20814; tel. toll-free (US only) 800 621-5483; (001) 301-961-5940; www.members.aol.com/biobrite/bbhome.htm

Light masks – (*produce flashing red light.*)
LightMask; tel. 0870 516 8143; www.lightmask.com or www.light-therapy.com

RelaxEase (*sold elsewhere as Relaxmate)* from Tools for Exploration, 9755 Independence Avenue, Chatsworth, CA 91311-4318; tel. 888 748-6657; International: (001) 818 885-9090), www.toolsforexploration.com

Magnets
Ladycare, LadyCare Health Products Ltd, 24 Emery Road, Brislington, Bristol BS4 5PF; order no. 08000 838 645; www.ladycarehealth.com

Nutricentre
Food supplements, herbal remedies, essential oils, etc:
The Hale Clinic, 7 Park Crescent, London W1N 3HE; www.nutricentre.com

Pelvic toner
('*Vaginal trainer*'); Natural Woman Ltd, 86 Shirehampton Road, Stoke Bishop, Bristol BS9 2DR, UK; tel. 0117 968 7744; www.pelvictoner.co.uk

Phyto Soya Vaginal Gel
Arkopharma, 7 Redlands Centre, Redlands, Coulsdon, Surrey CR5 HT; tel. 020 8763 1414

Rubber cup
'The Keeper'; tel. 0117 985 1646; www.menses.co.uk

Vaginal cones
Aquaflex; freephone (UK only) 0808 100 2890; www.aquaflexcones.com

Yeastguard pessaries
For stockists, tel. 0121 433 3727

index